THE TRUTH ABOUT CHRONIC PAIN

BY

Dr. Alex Tam

The truth about Chronic Pain.

Copyright © 2021 by Dr. Alex Tam

Table of Contents

Introduction

As you can probably tell from the cover, this is a book about pain and also what role chiropractic plays in relation to it. Chronic pain is a nuisance that many of us deal with and yet not many of us are told much about it beyond taking a pill to control it or that we would eventually need surgery. Chronic pain is so much more complicated than that, with many factors contributing to it including, but absolutely not limited to, structural misalignments, inflammation, nutritional deficiencies, and stress. It is important to look at chronic pain as a symptom with a root cause, one that will not be fixed by a pill or maybe even surgery. It is also prudent to note there is not any one thing that can "cure" your health problem; your BODY does the healing. You can do many things to help that process along but ultimately, your body's intelligence does all the healing.

For something that has been around for so long, not many people truly know and understand the origin and the purpose of chiropractic beyond post accident care and its role in helping with back pain. One of the purpose of this book is to look into the field that is chiropractic as well has how it is used to help chronic pain. I also wanted to give both my patients as well as those who may be skeptical about chiropractic look at the logic behind this science. Chiropractic is a science and a precise one at that. If more medical doctors come to realize the benefits of proper chiropractic care, they too may find themselves referring patients they once thought could only be treated by prescription drugs and surgery into the non-evasive, gentle care of their local chiropractor.

In writing this book, I sought out the experience of other chiropractors so that I could add their research and expertise to my own in creating a well-rounded publication that would inform and educate my readers not only on some common contributors to chronic pain and the role chiropractic plays in helping manage it, but also on how to live a life centered in wellness. I found out that although we have our textbooks and clinical trial summaries, there is not a whole lot out there for the average "lay" person. I wanted an easy to read summary of various medical conditions and lifestyle choices that can help you better understand the holistic management of chronic pain and the chiropractic way of life.

One of the many purposes of this book is to educate and inform readers about the part chiropractic plays in a life of good mental and physical health and wellness. I feel like this is something that is never talked about. When you hear about chiropractic, the majority of it centers on how it can help with back pain. While that is true, chiropractic is so much more than that. Chiropractic, along with other lifestyle choices and good habits, can create a sense of wellness that goes beyond fighting disease and illness. Like the saying goes, "An ounce of prevention is worth a pound of the cure." Chiropractic care, in conjunction with a healthy conscious lifestyle, can play a vital role in truly feeling well in every sense of the word. It is a compilation of common conditions I've seen in practice and answers to common questions I have been asked by patients over a decade of practice all under one cover.

So what can you expect from this book? Common sense! We as a culture are so inundated with thinking that in order for something to work, it has to be complicated. Nothing could be further from the truth. If it's complicated it won't be used. It's that simple. Look at the personal computer revolution. Up until the introduction of the Apple computer, computers were feared, and no one used them -- not the masses at least. Then along came Steve Jobs, who revolutionized the personal computer industry through simplicity. It is time to revolutionize the health industry by creating concepts that are easy to understand and most importantly, are applied because simplicity is the key. If it's not simple you will have all the excuses in the world to not use them.

Keeping the concept of simplicity in mind, this book is going to talk about things that are simple to do that can make a huge difference in your overall health. Goals and accomplishments must be perceived as being doable or we aren't going to even attempt them. The processes discussed in this book will be full of easy, doable processes that can make a world of a difference in your life.

We unfortunately believe that we can change our lives overnight. The truth is that we can change our *mind* overnight, but our body doesn't change that quickly. This is because whatever it was that created the condition of our body didn't happen overnight or even take one or two weeks; it took a lifetime. So if you want to change your health for the good, you must look at the healing factor differently. Look at it as an ongoing process that you begin today.

What you need to do to get something out of this book is begin by opening your mind. They say the mind is like a parachute, and it won't work if it's not opened. You must have an open mind to try out new ideas, especially those actions that may not be as widely accepted by the mainstream population.

We as a society fear change. Yet we continue on the path that has brought us to the condition of health that we now experience. Somehow we expect in our minds that even staying on the same path can yield different results than the last time we started down it. That is the definition of insanity: doing the same things over and over and expecting different results. Be curious with trying new things. Be open to new possibilities. Be open to doing something and it not "working at first." That's okay. You'll just try again.

It's a myth that in order for us to be successful, we must succeed the first time at something. Life is a process. It is an experience. We must go through life with the courage that we will sometimes fall or sometimes fail. The most important thing that we can do is to get back up. That is the key to success: Get back up when you fall.

Open your heart and open your mind and begin to explore the possibilities of a new life. The life I am talking about is a life with more energy, more vitality, and most of all, a life full of HEALTH!

Stumbling Blocks to Success

This book is only as good as what you can get out of it. Fear of change can be one of the biggest obstacles that can prevent you from getting the most out of this book. It rids you of desire to improve and justifies why you continue to do what you do. Don't let fear hold you back: it can rob you of your health and well being.

"I can't do this because [insert excuse here]." Does this sound familiar? Excuses will dry up your motivation more than anything out there. Don't make any more excuses. There is a saying, "It's not the situation that you are in that holds you back; it is the excuses that you use to justify the situation." Don't let excuses stand between you and good health!

Many patients tell me, "I'm tired of feeling this; I don't want to feel pain anymore." Or they may tell me, "I don't want to feel tired anymore." Problem is that tell me what they *don't* want to feel. I explain to them that if they focus all their energy on how they don't want to feel, how can they concentrate on what you *do* want? Focus on what you want, not on what you don't want. That is the key!

It is my hope that by reading this book you too can come to the decision that chiropractic care is a part of health care and wellness that everyone needs -- not just those with back problems. It can provide you with a proactive approach to your health. It can also open the body up to its full self-healing potential. Not too many doctors and pharmacists would dare make that claim. I invite you to read on and learn more about this proven scientific method of wellness and all that chiropractic encompasses.

The Simplicity Philosophy

Bottom line to good health and a system of managing it that you can use for a lifetime is simplicity. You must grab on to things that can work. Simple plans work. All you need is the confidence in yourself to implement the following information. Then you will find yourself making huge gains within your health.

Phenomenal healing powers are within you waiting to be unleashed. The key is to focus on the wins, and not get distracted by the setbacks. You will get them; we all will. This is the reality.

All of the principles you are going to learn in this book are based on laws of nature. They are not some kind of magical, cool sounding approach that contradicts simple common sense. They are quite simply the laws of life or perhaps you prefer to think of them as the laws of nature.

What you are going to learn here are the same principles that farmers abide by. They call it "The law of the farm." Basically, it is a natural law that affects us all, but too many people live by the effect of this law rather than abide over it. They let what happens control them instead of controlling what happens. You must understand that there are many theories out there and many have strong merit. But what good are they if you don't take action and are not consistent?

One example is the yo-yo weight loss and gain cycle which results from diet fads in this country. It alone is creating such a level of disease that it's driving health care costs through the roof. We must change something now!

Technology's Role in Health Care

Sure technology has had a great impact on healthcare. We see the evolution of the x-ray and ultrasound that lets us see into the body what we could only approximate before. In this book, however, you will learn about a technology that is so simple to use that it will blow you away. You see that health should not be complicated. Anyone trying to complicate health is trying to get you to be dependent on them so you rely on them solely, and you forget your own judgment.

That has been the problem within the medical profession for some time. We have abided by the opinions of our healthcare professionals and their latest technologies, but it has brought us no more health than we expected. As a matter of fact, we in the United States fail miserably as a society according to the World Health Organization (WHO).

The WHO reports that the U.S. ranks 37th out of 200 countries in terms of quality of individual health and wellness. To put that into perspective, Columbia is ranked 39th. How can we accept such mediocre results from a country that spends more dollars on "health care" than any other country in the world?

What we are doing is simply not working. Innovation is at the heart of this book. No more complex strategies; we are going to get to the simple, bare bones concepts that you can immediately use in your everyday life and that can truly make a difference in your life.

Break away from the old and decide today for yourself that you are going to use a technology that will truly make a difference in your life. You deserve it, and those around you deserve someone who comes to the table alive, refreshed, energetic, and not just a partial representation of themselves. You deserve to reach the full you at your greatest potential! It should not be an option; this is your birthright.

Why do we need to think outside the box? This expression has been used for many years now and although it sounds cliché, it holds true more today than ever. We must change our paradigm from disease care, which we are clearly in, to a preventative care way of looking at health. It's the most cost effective way of taking care of our bodies.

This is not a new concept in other areas, so why should it be so underutilized when it comes to health? The automotive companies have known about it since cars were invented. They are well aware that if you give your car preventative care such as periodic tune ups and oil changes they will last longer. It's that simple.

So the key is to trim the fat from our health care. I believe the best way to do that is not to rely on symptoms. If you wait until there are symptoms, most often you are too late. You will learn more about this later in the book, but please keep that concept in mind.

The tests and processes we are using to determine health are not showing the consequences of our diets of ten years ago. It doesn't show what is going on with our arteries from the stand point of what the food we consume today is going to do to our arteries 5 or 10 years from now. Insanity has crippled this health care system, and we must do something about this now, before it's too late. If we continue at this rate in 50 years we have the unfortunate opportunity of bankrupting this country due to health care costs. Costs have gone through the roof for HMO's and other insurance plans, and it is predicted that within 5 – 10 years health care deductibles will reach an annual level of more than $5,000 per person. That is ridiculous. You can do your part to change this. We all can when we approach our own health and that of our families in a preventative, proactive manner.

Disclaimer

Important Information for the Reader

This information presented in this book has been compiled from my clinical experience and research. It is offered as a view of the relationship between diet, exercise, emotions, and health. This book is not intended for self diagnosis or treatment of disease, nor is it a substitute for the advice and care of a licensed health care provider.

This book is intended solely to help you make better judgements concerning your long-term health goals. If you are experiencing health problems, you should consult a qualified physician immediately. Remember early examination and detection are important to successful treatment of all diseases.

Chapter 1

Appreciating the Marvel of Human Life

Before I discuss anything else, I want to take this chapter to appreciate this thing called human life, to appreciate the astounding way in which our human body works. I am not talking about something mystical. Instead, I'm asking you to think about the complexities of our body and to marvel about how we exist in the first place. Bottom line: OUR BODIES ARE AMAZING!

Just think about it: our body made of billions and billions of cells working in sync with each other, the heart that beats untiringly 100, 000 times a day, our breath and senses which send millions of signals each day, blood vessels extending thousands of miles and yet at the end of the day not a single breakdown. The key to changing our life is by first appreciating it.

Everything is marvelous about the way we take shape from day one. Our brain is the first organ that starts forming; Then it is covered by the bony shield we call a skull in adults and the our spinal cord, the powerful information highway, starts developing. Only once the central computing and information highway is ready do the other body parts, including the other organs, start taking shape. The autonomic nervous system takes over the control of our internal organs, ensuring that heart beats as intended and digestive juices are secreted as required.

This isn't quite Anatomy 101 but we can still see how intricate the body truly is. You can see the importance of the nervous system and how it controls the functioning of each and every cell, playing a crucial role in health maintenance by responding to every challenge.

However, if our nervous system somehow fails to respond to these daily challenges suitably, the balance is broken and what happens when our bodies are out of balance? You got it... it leads to disease. So how can we make sure this doesn't happen?

Remember this: **Doctor's don't cure, drugs do not cure....because the body cures itself.**

A true healer acknowledges this fact and truly appreciates the flow of the healing power inside each of us.

Thank your body in serving you in such a beautiful manner and respect and appreciate the abilities of your body and treat it as the most precious thing you have ever owned because it truly is. You only get one body. Treat it well.

Innate Intelligence and the Body's Functions

As I already mentioned earlier, the body starts with a single cell. But how does that single cell transform into a whole body?

It isn't exactly magical but it is nothing short of miraculous. It does so in a process chiropractors have been calling *Innate Intelligence* for more than a century. Innate Intelligence is something that is created at the moment of your conception; it flows through your body. It is what makes your body function in a way it should be functioning without a glitch. It operates automatically. It does everything from maintaining your heart rhythm to keeping your skin supple. Let's take a deeper dive into how innate intelligence in body works.

The lungs

Lungs are another brilliant example of Innate Intelligence at work. The primary function of lungs is to keep your body oxygenated and to remove carbon dioxide and other wastes of metabolism. During inhalation, our rib cage expands to allow maximum air inside, while during exhalation the rib cage becomes smaller to push out the air. Ribs are quite dynamic and muscles between them are flexible, allowing air to flow in and out of the lungs.

Though automatic, respiration is a highly regulated process, enabling us to breathe about 20000 times a day and works continually under the supervision of the autonomic nervous system.

The Skin

Skin is not there just to provide the cover for the body. In fact, it is the largest organ of our body amounting to about 16 percent of total body weight. Apart from protection, it helps to maintain body temperature, removes excess water, salt, and toxins.

Skin is the first line of defense for our internal organs from every imaginable danger, be it infection or ultraviolet rays. Skin even converts sun rays to vitamin D which helps to maintain healthy bones.

Skin also plays a vital role in communication, sensation, expression of emotions, and even sexual attraction. It is made up of three layers called epidermis, dermis, and the hypodermis.

The Digestive System

Digestion starts in the mouth from the moment you eat. Saliva contains enzymes that start breaking down the food while chewing food is considered part of digestion. From there, food reaches the stomach while passing through the pipe called the esophagus. The stomach has juices that can help digest and break down the food. From there, the broken down food moves into the intestines to be absorbed and the leftovers ultimately excreted. Movement of food in the digestive system happens due to a rhythmic wave movement called peristalsis. It is an action that is similar to squeezing a ball from one end of a soft tube to the other end. Peristalsis is a brilliant example of Innate Intelligence at work.

The Eyes

Despite their small size, eyes are a very important sensory organ, with millions of cells that provide the sense of sight. Although eyes can perceive only red, yellow, blue, and black, they can differentiate between 300 trillion colors!

Sitting in the bony socket of the skull, each eye has a lens to focus light on the sensor called the retina. The retina sends visual information to the brain with the help of optical nerves. The small colored portion in the center of the eyes called the iris, controls the amount of light that can enter inside the eye. In bright light the pupil contracts, while in low light conditions they dilate to allow more light into the eyes.

Eyes are protected by eyelids and eyelashes. They blink on a regular interval to keep the upper layer of eyes moist.

All these activities in the eyes happen automatically due to innate intelligence.

The Muscles

There are whopping 650 muscles in our body, making all of our movements possible. They are made to do the most complicated tasks like picking small objects with tweezers to more robust tasks like running a marathon. Muscles also help to protect the internal organs.

To perform any tasks, muscles must work in synchronization with various other organs. Moving from one place to another involves communication between muscles, ears, eyes and brain. This internal communication happens by using the information highway called our nervous system.

When our muscles and joints are moving, all the information about actions, movement,and location is being transmitted to the brain at a subconscious level. This communication is controlled by innate intelligence.

If a person starts talking to you, you automatically turn your head, eyes and start listening. It is the Innate Intelligence of your body that makes all this possible by controlling the minor muscular movements at all times. Our balance and movement will become sluggish if even one small muscle fails to perform as required. Thus, the brain has to keep correcting the movement at all times.

The Skeletal System

Without bones we would be just an enormous blob with no shape or structure. We would not be able to stand or walk. Without bones, we would be just a pile of skin, muscles, and guts.

Our skeletal system is made up of 206 bones, designed to be strong, and to protect our body. At birth we have 300 bones, but as we grow many of them fuse together.

Bones have many functions. The spinal vertebrae not only protect the information highway that is the spinal cord but also help us to stand erect and walk upright. Bones also protect the delicate internal organs. Just consider the skull. It's like a strong helmet safeguarding our brain. The rib cage protects our heart and lungs.

Unlike the common perception that bones are cold and inert, they are in fact, very dynamic. Bones are made of a hard layer for providing strength and cells that help them grow and repair. That is why if you have ever broken your arm or leg, it heals.

Apart from mechanical support and protection, bones are also responsible for producing red and white blood cells. Red blood cells are responsible for carrying oxygen to body tissues, while white blood cells are the part of the immune system, thus helping to protect our body from infections and diseases.

Once Again,... The Nervous System Is Amazing!

We once again return to discuss the system that controls our majestic body- the nervous system. It consists of the brain, spinal cord and peripheral nerves. The brain is the main computing center that sends signals to various parts of the body, performing billions of operations, yet consuming merely around ten watts of energy. The spinal cord is the information "Superhighway," that is responsible for distributing all the information. Spinal nerves are the exit points of the highway.

The nervous system is operated by the Innate Intelligence that is vital for the functioning of every cell. Most of the time, it efficiently performs its tasks to ensure that the body works in tandem for proper health. Any disruption in communication between the body parts and the brain would lead to either pain or a loss of function. It is like a disruption in the telephone line which compromises communication between two parties.

For optimal health, it is vital that our nervous system is working correctly all the time to maintain hundred percent communication throughout the body. As you can see in this chapter, our body is made up of various systems that operate in synchronization with each other to ensure optimal health under the guidance of Innate Intelligence.

Action Steps:

1. Evaluate your own life and amazing body. How has your body responded to sickness and stress?

2. Take time for thanks and gratefulness for your Innate Intelligence and amazing body.

3. Ask yourself, "Do I have a plan to take care of my amazing body? Am I proactive or am I waiting for problems to take action?"

Chapter 2

What Is "Health"?

S uppose that I were to ask you to define the term "health." What kind of answer would you give me? There is a general opinion and consensus that good health is: (1) feeling "fine," or (2) when everything is working okay, or (3) when there is an absence of pain.

All of these definitions are partial and are far from complete. Taber's medical dictionary defines health as, "A condition in which all functions of the body and mind are normally active." The World Health Organization defines health as a state of complete physical, mental or social well-being and not merely the absence of disease or infirmity. So the next question to ask is how does one quantify health? In a sense then, health is equal to balance. How do you determine balance? What are the determining factors in the balancing equation? To answer this we must first ask, what comprises the overall scheme of health? Also, what kind of an overall gauge can be used to reflect back on the quality of health we experience or lack there of?

In order to get to the core of good health you need to start at the cellular level. The balancing act begins there. You see, the quality of your life is based on the quality of the life of your cells. Considering the fact that you are comprised of over 70 trillion cells, you can assume that when those cells are working optimally in perfect harmony with each other, you will have health. But again how does one quantify this?

Now if health equals balance, then we can state that the opposite of health, which is not disease, but rather dis-ease meaning a lack of balance or ease. It can also be said that the cells are not functioning correctly.

Raymond Francis, a chemist and graduate of MIT, believes through his research that there is only one reason in which disease is created. That reason is simply due to cells not functioning properly. When you think about that statement, it makes sense. Now there are only two reasons why cells do not function appropriately. They are:

1. Cells are not receiving proper nutrition and/or
2. Cells are not eliminating their toxicity produced by the normal functioning of the cell.

Now there are at the root many reasons why these cells can become dysfunctional. Those reasons are:

- Lack of appropriate levels of oxygen
- Lack of nutrients
- The inability to eliminate waste
- Improper nerve impulse to the cell

To begin to understand this process let us quickly visit the stages of health. When one is conceived, we are given as a birthright the ability to express health effortlessly. However if there is a disturbance in the intimate relationship between the nervous system and the rest of the body, you will lose your efficient ability to express health.

As we age, we experience the effects of the years initially only through a microscopic inspection. Long before we feel the effects of age, our cells are beginning to experience changes. Cells are beginning to replicate less efficiently, and then one day we transition from the anabolic phase of life, which means that sufficient cells are replacing those that have just died, to a phase of catabolic metabolism, in which we have more cells that are dying than are being replaced. When we enter the catabolic stage, we must do everything within our power to slow it down.

To better understand the process of health, it helps to understand the phases of health. The first phase is one of perfect balance or homeostasis. This is optimal health where everything is working the way it was designed to work. However, as we age, we begin to encounter emotional, physical, and chemical stresses in our lives to the point where we will enter into a phase of imbalance, lack of ease, or dis-ease. Health can easily be regained in this phase as long as we refocus our efforts on finding the cause of what brought us initially on that path of imbalance. If that is achieved, then we can regain a state of balance.

However, if this phase is not dealt with appropriately, then we enter into a phase of discomfort, and dis-ease. This phase can have with it associated levels of pain, but not in all cases. Sometime there are no visible or felt symptoms. If we stay in this phase for any real amount of time, we begin to have dis-ease of more than one cell. It begins to affect thousands and thousands of cells, to the point of reaching into the body's tissues. Left further without a reversal of the dis-ease, then it enters into a larger group of tissues which would then be affecting organs. It then moves onto systems, and then ultimately it affects the entire being, and we then die.

I'm not proposing that we can live forever. I am however saying that 90% of our medical expense is spent during the last 10% of our lives. People are no longer dying of natural causes. The majority of deaths in this country are related to degenerative processes. When one can minimize that process one can live a longer, higher quality of life.

Therefore, the key to overall health is to correctly determine the appropriate factors involved in health. This means managing health at the cellular level. Health is a consequence of choices one has made or not made.

A Doctor's Approach to Health

Imagine going to a doctor when you had nothing wrong with you. Your blood pressure was fine, your cholesterol was reasonable, your weight was appropriate for your age and height. What if at this visit you told the doctor that all you wanted to do was maintain this? Hopefully he or she would say, "great," but they may not be able to offer you much more in the way of maintenance than to say, "keep on doing whatever you are doing." The point here is that that kind of advice would only work for so long. That is because the medical system is at best designed for the early detection of disease, but not for the prevention.

How would you react to a mechanic who told you that all you need to do for your car is bring it in and have the oil changed when the car starts to give you problems? We all know what that would do, don't we? We know what the consequences of not getting an oil change on time does to our car, which incidentally we will only have for 10 years at best, and yet we don't always give our one and only body the same kind of preventative care.

Why do we put so little effort into maintaining our bodies? That is because most people believe that there is a magic pill that will solve all of our problems. Again, no medicine has ever, ever cured anyone. The body does the healing; it happens no other way.

The birth of medicine could be attributed to the time when Robert Koch postulated the germ theory in 1860. Once this discovery took place, it was therefore emphasized and widely believed that microbes were the cause of disease. It was also widely accepted that the key to health was to destroy those foreign enemies.

This theory has resulted in the overuse of antibiotics to the point that we are now dealing with super-strains of bacteria and viruses. These microbes are becoming more and more resistant to all of the antibiotics originally created to fight them off.

Alternative Health Options

People today are becoming more and more aware of alternatives. They are sick and tired of being sick and tired and they want options. They want to know why they are sick or why they are feeling a certain way. They are sick and tired of hearing obscure explanations on what they have and why taking a "magic pill" will solve all their problems.

We are getting smarter. It's true! In the United States in the year 2001, there were more visits to Alternative Health Care practitioners than traditional allopathic medical doctors. It may have started with the baby boomers who wanted to create and maintain health, not just mask their problems with drugs and surgery. We are not being attacked by the flu. We are not innocent victims being chosen by microbes. We are, in fact, creating the very environment for these bacteria and viruses to feast upon: a body that is full of toxicity -- the perfect environment in which bacteria and viruses thrive.

Anyone can change their attitude and approach to health. If you continue to look at your body the same way you have in the past, you will continue to get what you have gotten in the past. However, if you want to change things, start with your mindset. You must prioritize your health as not something that should be tolerated, but something that must be maintained and even improved. In life, it seems we only do consistently that which we find important enough to make a priority. It is important, therefore, to look at your health as something that is so important that it becomes top priority.

To make your health a priority you must realize that there are a variety of different choices we make everyday that can be categorized into two broad areas: Doing things that are important and urgent; and doing things that are important and not urgent.

Everything in your life that adds meaning to your life and fulfillment to it, such as spending time with your family, working out, eating the right foods, spending quality time with your significant other, are all under the category of things that are important but not urgent. In order for you to create the highest level of health possible, you must consistently focus on doing things in the area of health that are important for you.

The question to ask yourself is, "What can I do today to start on a path of wellness?" I recommend that my patients make the changes that are very easy and simple to do. For example, I had a patient who had not exercised in many, many years. I asked her if she could spend 5 minutes a day just stretching. Of course that sounded very easy to do. Before long, that 5 minute stretch turned into 10 minutes. Next, she realized that the stretching really felt good and added some light resistance to her routine with some hand weights. By the end of a month, she had added cardio to the routine and was up to a half hour of exercising. It felt so good that the habit was one she intended on maintaining.

You see, once you create a habit, you can expand upon it, but you will set yourself up for failure if you start too big. The most important thing that I want you to get out of this chapter is the subtle consequences our choices have on our health. There are small decisions we make everyday that can make the difference between being completely well or not.

If you would like to test out this theory for yourself, I have an assignment for you! First, get yourself a health journal. It can be any small notebook that you can keep with you. Next, write down the following on the inside cover or first page of your journal:

"I hereby grant myself permission to bring my health to the highest level I was meant to experience, by nurturing myself, by taking care of myself, and by forgiving myself as I would a loved one. I declare today, a day that I will never forget, for it is the day that my life and health was changed forever."

Your health journal should begin with a list of goals. These can be categorized as physical, mental and spiritual. You may want to eat better, so be specific and list the types of foods you will avoid to obtain better health. If you want to learn a new skill or improve a relationship, list specific actions you can take and over which you have complete control. The more specific you are the more successful you will be.

Each day, record in your journal or notebook the small steps you have taken. Record even your set backs and shortcomings because those will help you see the progress you are making over time.

How Can Chiropractic Care Effect Your Health?

The biggest way chiropractic can help you is by number one not focusing on symptoms, but rather on the body's ability to regain health. If you always chase symptoms, you will never truly regain your body's health potential. You will always be days or months away from your next symptom, and you will be focused on relieving those symptoms as quickly as possible.

Being under chiropractic care allows you to change your perception of going to the doctor only when there is a problem to going to the chiropractor because you don't want to have any problems in the future.

Where would we be if we had a health care system in which the doctors were only paid based on how healthy their patients are? Sound crazy? That's exactly what is happening in Japan. Doctors get paid based on how healthy their patients are. It does not impress me whatsoever, when a doctor says that it's a good thing that you came in because we just found some major problems in you, and we need to go in immediately for a bypass, or something equally invasive. Problems like that just don't appear out of nowhere. It takes years and years for conditions to develop and get to that point. Again we have technology within the medical community that emphasizes early detection at best and very little, if any, prevention.

You can't just blame the doctors here either. It is the responsibility of each individual to care for themselves and to take action to prevent disease. It is the responsibility of every parent to see that their children are on a path of good, life long health through preventative care.

How Can Chiropractic Be A Strategy To Attain Health?

The science of chiropractic is in and of itself a fundamental strategy for good health. When you are under chiropractic care, you work to reduce any stress or strain around the spine which in turn could affect the body's ability to adapt to all that is thrown its way.

You see, if there is any kind of interference within or surrounding the nervous system it causes dis-ease or creates a situation where you are not completely well. Often that interference can't be felt. There may no pain or pressure at all to tell you something isn't right. Rather the only thing you experience from this is the effects of it. Sadly, it may take months or even years for the symptoms to manifest themselves.

This might be easier to understand if you use the example of breast cancer. Did you know that it takes years to create enough density within the breast tissue in order to see a tumor growth via X-ray? By that time it may be too late.

Chiropractic does not emphasize waiting for something to go wrong, and then coming in as the hero to only remove the symptom, doing very little about the actual cause of the problem. It focuses on maintaining your natural state of wellness at an optimal level of existence, so that you are at the highest level neurologically speaking.

Think about it this way: if you applied the same rationale to your life in every aspect, would it make your life better or richer, or would it make it worse? If you applied the preventative model to your finances, what would it do? If you applied it to your relationship with your spouse, what would that do? All the areas of your life would see a marked improvement. You would no longer be waiting for things to get to the point of being urgent. You would be proactive instead of reactive. You are prioritizing your health as being important while not waiting for a crisis to make changes.

How Chiropractic Can Change Your Life

Information and Empowerment. You see, with information and empowerment you can truly make a difference in your life. Here is a summary of the key factors needed to sustain health.

The first aspect of the system involves beliefs. The mind is a powerful tool in attaining your goals. In other words, you must believe in things that you want to have happen.

Next is to understand the importance of exercise. You must exercise, no if, ands, or buts about it. It doesn't end with you getting physical activity at work, or that you already chase the kids around the house, and already work in the garden. All of these activities are a good start to movement, but do not constitute a real workout. You must have a cardiovascular workout for health – one that challenges and works your heart. Remember your heart is a muscle and it needs to pump a lot of blood through your entire body every day for a very long time. You must challenge it so it can be as strong as possible.

The third aspect of this equation is the importance of breathing correctly. You must provide oxygen to the tissues of the body. If you don't, you will have problems because they will suffocate. Oxygen supplies and nourishes not only the lungs, but every cell within the body. The lungs are just the clearinghouse.

The fourth important factor is drinking water. This is necessary in order to flush out toxins from the body. After all your body is 75% water; not 75% coffee, or tea, or soda. These drinks just give you an illusion of energy. There is no sustaining power behind any of them, even though the caffeine addict may object to this statement.

The next fundamental truth relates to greens. Most people do not understand the magnitude of the importance of greens. Eating enough green, leafy vegetables each week is one of the most powerful things you can do for yourself. Think about this to understand why plants are so necessary to good health. When plants are outside, they convert light into energy, in the process known as photosynthesis. Through this amazing process, we are able to literally consume energy through the plants.

Most importantly, you must consume some raw vegetables, or you are totally defeating the purpose. Raw plants contain the necessary enzymes that are often destroyed by over cooking. Enzymes are vital to good health.

The next nutrient that you need to have is antioxidants. Antioxidants allow you to minimize the ravaging effects of free radicals that are within us and increase in number as we age. Free radicals are produced in times of stress, during injury, or during chemical processes that are taking place due to the consumption of processed foods. Free radicals left to roam can cause damage right at the cellular level. Damaged cells lead to a lowered immune system and increase the likelihood of infection and disease.

The next dietary items you need to have are fats and oils. Fats are needed to assure that your body has sufficient levels of oil to make the cell membrane of the cell. This outer layer of the cell is made of a double layer called a biphospholipid layer.

The problem with fats and oils in the diet is that many of us consume too much or the wrong type of fats. According to researchers, the average person is deficient in correct oil consumption by up to 90%! That is staggering considering the connection between low levels of essential oils in our diets and cardiovascular disease and the resulting list of degenerative disorders. So, believe it or not, oils are by far the best preventative measure that you can take.

The last pro-active step that you need to take is to maintain a healthy nervous system. Think about this for a moment. If you were consuming everything that I recommended, and yet your nervous system was not functioning properly, how would the brain tell the cells what to do with the nutrients it just received? How would the brain contact the cell to let it know when to remove waste?

Consider this research from a professor by the name of Professor Tzu. He claims that pressure put on a nerve with the weight of only a dime can interfere with normal transmission of impulse by up to 60%! It is staggering how little pressure it takes to reduce your body's own ability to send corrective, healing messages by so much.

Chapter 3

The Nervous System - Central to Good Health

Understanding the nervous system is an important part of understanding chiropractic as it is the foundation in which chiropractic was built on.

When we were first conceived, the first thing created in all of us was the brain. Next, it was carefully encased in a bony hard substance called the cranium (skull). Afterwards, the spinal cord, an extension of the brain was created, and that too was encased in a protective layer called the vertebrae or spinal column.

The next part to be developed in-utero was the spinal nerve roots, which are extensions of the spinal cord. Ultimately, those spinal nerve roots create spinal nerves which are surrounded by embryonic tissue. The brain is then stimulated by the embryonic tissue via the super highway called the nervous system. It was then and only then, that the other systems in the body developed.

You see, the nervous system is what controls all the systems in the body. If you were to look up nervous system in the Webster's Dictionary, you would find it defined as the following: "The master control system of the body that controls all other systems of the body."

The nervous system consists of three different areas. The first is the brain. It is the originator of the messages that are needed to be distributed to all the cells, tissues, organs, and systems of the body.

The second part of the nervous system is the spinal cord. Think of it as the super highway of the nervous system. It is a complex system which has routes to every aspect of our body.

The third part of the nervous system are the spinal nerves. Think of this as an exit off the main highway. Without these exits, you can never really get to a specific destination.

The brain weighs only 3 pounds. It needs only the energy of a 10 watt bulb, yet the functions of the brain are truly staggering. The brain is so complete and complex in its function that you would need two buildings the size of the Empire State Building to house today's technology that would rival the power of the brain!

Let me explain further. The brain can perform billions of operations simultaneously. Billions! A computer can only perform a few tasks at a time. A computer can perform the tasks at astounding speeds, but it can only perform a few functions at a time. Therefore, in order to have the computer be able to replicate the full capacity of the nervous system, you would need a massive system enabling the computer to perform complex tasks; billions of them at the same time. That is why the nervous system is called the master control system of the body. It controls all other systems. Without it, you could not survive.

Here is another way to emphasize the importance of the nervous system. If you cut the nerve to the lungs, how would the lung know what to do? Think of the lung as an appliance, and the spinal cord is the circuit. If the circuit breaker isn't allowing energy to flow into the outlet that supplies the appliance, the appliance is not going to work. It's the same with the cells, tissues, organs, and systems of the body.

The Workings of the Nervous System

Intelligence flows through every cell in the body. This intelligence is referred to by chiropractors as Innate Intelligence. Without this intelligence, there would be no order and no collaboration within our body.

There is an internal divine guidance that guides all the functions of the body. It knows exactly what substance to produce at the exact time needed. The nerve connections within our body are truly staggering. In the brain alone, there are more possible connections than there are possible combinations of phone lines within the Unites States. Just imagine that number!

So what prevents our body from doing its thing? What prevents this splendid orchestra from playing its tune called health?

Interference with the nervous system can have serious complications. Think about this for a moment. If I'm on a phone and I'm giving you very detailed instructions on how to get from point A to point B, and all of a sudden your phone begins to break up, will you be able to accurately get the directions you need to get to your destination? Now, this is not because you are incompetent. It is simply due to the fact that there was a break in your communication with me.

The key is to maintain 100 % communication within every aspect of the body. The researchers are just beginning to understand that there are mechanisms within our body that are trying to communicate something very important. One example is fever. At first, fever was regarded as something that needed to be stopped. We now know that it is designed to throw off the foreign invaders.

How did we react to fevers just 10 years ago? We pushed fever reducing substances down our children's throats, and we bought into the belief that they needed to be stopped. There are so many similar examples where information is conflicting and confusing. That is why I'm writing this book -- to at least give you a basic understanding of your body and what you can do immediately to bring it the next level. You have a very sophisticated body which requires a sophisticated understanding on how to provide it with the essential care it needs.

If the entire nervous system is fully functioning and fully interactive, with all the cells, tissues, organs, and other systems in the body, then the body can effectively and efficiently respond appropriately to changing conditions in the body. However, if the nervous system is not functioning properly, then you will find that it will create an imbalance, or lack of ease also called dis-ease.

The mindset that we have in regards to our bodies must be changed. Do we just get by in a world where our body is assaulted by the living of everyday life, or is life a miracle, and the body that I am in the temple of my soul? Do we have reverence for our bodies? Again this book is a wake up call for you to realize that there is so much in all of us to stimulate health -- so much potential. Unfortunately, most of the time, through ignorance, that potential remains untapped.

In coming chapters you will realize that our bodies can be the most amazing source of super immuno-stimulation and yet it can also be the greatest source of disease creation. The great researcher Gary Null, has advocated that health can be broken down into 25% nutrition, 25% exercising, and a whopping 50% mental attitude. If we have certain expectations and we believe them with certainty, those expectations will manifest in the physical world. In other words, you truly become what you think about, good or bad! What we must remember is that the intelligence that created us at conception still flows through every cell in our body today, and we must honor that.

I tell my patients that the body is providing us with signals, and we cannot ignore those signals. Again, I will stress one thing: I or any other chiropractor, medical doctor, or naturopath do not cure anything or anyone! The body does the curing. Think about it.

The body can either be used in its amazing splendor or it can be abused, and if it is abused, you will suffer with the consequences. So if we are to attain incredible levels of health, we must first start with an equivalent level of gratitude for our body and respect for it. When you realize that you have a choice, to make this life what you want of it, to carve out of life what you want, to create a magical life full of passion, vibrancy, and possibility, then you must be grateful for what you have. There are so many things for which you can and should be grateful. The body that you are in right now is doing everything it can to support you at this very moment. It is there to serve you. So today I want you to decide that from now on, you will no longer look at your body as something that deserves a candy bar or a soda. Think of it as one of the finest, exotic cars in the world, one that deserves and should receive only the best fuel.

If you owned a $100,000 race horse, you would train it constantly. You would feed it the best food possible. Why? Because you paid all that money and you expect to get a return on your investment. Well what do you suppose you and your health are worth? How much would you be willing to pay for a liver transplant? How much for a kidney transplant? How much for a heart transplant? How much for your hearing? How much for your vision? Can you now see how valuable and priceless you really are?

Realize that you are a gift and that you are here for a reason. That you are here for a specific reason. You can't attain your heart's desires without the spark of energy derived from a true level of health and well being. Begin today with a new appreciation for your body and what true health can do for you.

The Spine

The primary component to chiropractic is, of course, the spine. It is the spine, which is made up of the spinal cord and vertebrae that is central to the science of chiropractic.

By giving you a little anatomy lesson on the spine, it will help you understand how and why chiropractic makes so much sense to those of us who have adopted this practice as our lifelong vocation.

The spinal column is a row of bones that encircle the spinal cord. The spinal cord is the central component of the central nervous system which transmits signals throughout the body. Some people assume that the spinal cord and nerves only transmit signals about touch and pain.

It is believed that the nerves signal the brain when you touch something hot, pain then registers in the brain and you quickly remove your hand from the iron. This much is true, but there is so much more information that the nervous system communicates to the brain and other organs in the body.

In chiropractic it is known that every area of the body is supplied with information that comes from the nerves. When there is no static or interference (in the form of subluxations (or misalignments)) in the message transmitted, every organ can function at its fullest capacity. That is the number one purpose of chiropractic – to remove static from the message signals and open the channels for the body to mend and heal using its own innate intelligence.

Regions of the Spine

The spine can be broken down into three key regions. There is the cervical spine, thoracic spine, and lumbar spine. There is also a fourth area referred to as the sacral region. The sacral region, however, only has two bones: the sacrum and the coccyx. These are at the bottom of the spine and extend into the pelvic area.

Within the top three regions of the spine, the vertebrae are all assigned numbers. So when there is a misalignment in a particular vertebra, the chiropractor may explain to the patient that there is a subluxation caused by the misalignment of the C4 vertebra. This would mean the 4th vertebra from the top, or the 4th vertebra in the cervical spine, is misaligned.

A patient who has a blockage or misalignment in the C4 vertebra could actually be seeing the doctor about their hay fever and not necessarily back pain. That is because the nerves that extend from the C4 vertebra are responsible for messages sent to the nose, lips, mouth, eustachian tube (ear canal), and mucous membranes. Often a misalignment here manifests itself as hay fever, postnasal drip, adenoid infections, and other upper respiratory symptoms. There can even be problems with hearing by a misalignment of the C4 vertebra!

Every nerve that extends from the spinal column is responsible for an organ, function, or performance of some part of the body. This includes the obvious organs such as the sensory capabilities of touch, which goes literally to every part of the body. A complete body map shows this radial effect. If you were to envision an outline of the body and create lines from the center where the spine would be located, drawn out to each extremity, then you can see how the nerves and protective vertebrae are assigned to those areas within the body. You can also see clearly, then, how if the vertebra meant to protect the nerve gets pushed out of place, even slightly, how that can have an impact on the nerve signals that go out from that region of the spine.

This idea of the vertebrae being labeled and the corresponding nerves reaching out to all areas of the body is not exclusive to chiropractic. The medical field also recognizes the anatomy and what it means to have something out of alignment. Where mainstream medicine and chiropractic differ, is in the way it is treated and in recognizing the full impact of the misalignment.

How the Spine Moves

The spine is able to bend and move and return to its "s"-like shape without incident or injury because of some of the soft tissue that works with the bony vertebrae. There are two types of soft tissue that are important in helping the spinal column protect the large central nerve, the spinal cord.

An inter-vertebral disc can be found between each vertebra. This disc helps absorb shock as the spine bends and twists during normal movement and activity. It also protects the vertebrae and spine from excessive shock. You don't think about that as you bend down to pick up a toy off the floor, because everything is in its proper place.

You can even bend and twist to one side to grasp the toy that slid under the chair. Still no problems. However, if you were to have a deterioration of that disc or if it were to have slipped out of place even a little, there could be a grinding of the bone and a pinching of a nerve, and you would feel pain.

This type of back injury or painful condition is probably the number one reason people visit a chiropractor. Luckily, there are so many more health reasons that keep them returning to the chiropractor to maintain their overall health.

The second type of tissue is the facet joint. This allows for limited movement of the spine. The facet joints regulate movement so that routine movements are restricted to the point that they will not injure the spinal cord. The body, with its innate ability to heal, was created in a way that protects the most vital organs. The ribs protect the heart and lungs. The skull protects the brain. Then there is the spinal column to protect the spinal cord.

Misaligned Vertebrae

Every nerve in the body that radiates from the spinal cord supplies important information to the area of the body for which it is responsible. The example of the C4 vertebra being out of alignment is just one of literally hundreds of slight misalignments that can interfere with the nerve signal, and result in some kind of ailment.

In the medical world, a patient visiting the doctor for indigestion or heartburn will almost immediately be prescribed some kind of antacid to ease those uncomfortable symptoms. For some people, this kind of quick fix may be okay for a while. After all, we all want to get rid of painful discomfort as quickly as possible. The problem with this treatment is that it doesn't cure the problem. It hardly even addresses the problem and certainly neglects the real cause of the problem. How can the body ever hope to heal itself if medications are momentarily quieting the symptoms?

Symptoms are there for a reason. The body, in its wisdom, has to let the brain know something isn't right. If we just quiet that inner voice with a medication, it's like telling someone to stop talking when they see you are about to get hit by a car. They are trying to give you an important message, but if you ignore it long enough, you will eventually have to deal with a much bigger problem.

When there is a symptom related to the stomach, it can often be traced back to the T6 vertebra. It is from this area that stomach problems and the body's ability to correct them transmit. The nerves in the T6 region could be experiencing some kind of interference. Removing that blockage through an adjustment of the spine will open up the lines of communication to the stomach and allow the problems in that region to be corrected naturally.

This simplified lesson on the anatomy of the spine is meant to illustrate the complex nature of the spinal column and the central nervous system. It is not quite as simple as explained here. There are so many minor misalignments that can impact one region of the body. Likewise, there are many different ways in which symptoms manifest themselves that it isn't always easy to pinpoint just what the real problem is. Back pain can often originate in the stomach and vice versa. Headaches can be the symptom for so many other ailments that may start out in a completely different area of the body. The complexities of this whole system is what chiropractors study for years so that they can perform the right diagnostic tests and begin the correct treatment for any specific ailment.

Chapter 4

Healthy Organs

To understand how to achieve health, we must understand the general role of the different parts of the body. This is not an exhaustive list, just a short summary of some of the most important parts.

The Heart

How is the heart such a miraculous muscle? Synchronicity could be a way of describing the heart. It is an elaborate mechanism of supplying the entire body with blood and one that marvels scientists to this day.

On average, your heart beats 100,000 times a day without you having to think about it. It doesn't take any time outs; it doesn't go on vacation. It does its job every second of the day. Also, on average the heart pumps over 6,000 quarts of blood a day through a network of vessels that span close to 60,000 miles throughout the body. In an average life span, the heart will beat over 1 billion times. The heart's valves are made up of tissue so delicate that they are thinner than tissue paper, yet this muscle is the strongest muscle in the human body.

It is important to remember that the heart is a muscle. A muscle that is not used will wither away and atrophy. When you go to bed, your heart rate goes down to conserve energy so as to rebuild and renew itself. All of this ingenuity and it only weighs between 9 and 11 ounces! The whole point of the heart is to pick up oxygen from the lungs and supply it throughout the body. It's that simple.

The Lungs

Twenty thousand breaths are taken every day without our conscious awareness of it. We breathe in and out to provide oxygen that constitutes around 300 gallons of air, or 90 gallons of pure oxygen. Our lungs are an amazing example of coordination at its finest. The lungs are needed to provide oxygen to the cells, in which the heart circulates the oxygenated blood thereafter. This process is done by allowing the diaphragm to contract causing the lungs to expand.

When you exhale, the relaxation of the muscles takes place, and the air is released out of the lungs. When you inhale, the diaphragm and muscles between the ribs (intercostals) contract. This allows the chest cavity to expand. This in turn causes the lungs to expand. This causes a change in the pressure inside the lungs allowing air to enter the lungs. When you exhale the diaphragm and intercostals muscles relax, causing the pressure inside the lungs to be greater than the pressure outside, which releases the air out of the body.

During this entire process of air exchange and release, the body, upon inspiration, absorbs the oxygen from the air through pulmonary capillaries, very small vessels located in the lung. Initially during inspiration, the hemoglobin in the red blood cells has attached to it carbon dioxide which must be released. This process takes place by oxygen entering into the air, which then binds with the hemoglobin of the red blood cell, causing the release of the carbon dioxide. The carbon dioxide is released through the lungs via expiration.

Thus the primary function of the lungs is to maintain high levels of oxygen within the blood, and to remove carbon dioxide from the blood. This amazing process is carefully regulated through an elaborate system within the nervous system. Within this system, every aspect of the breathing process is closely monitored at all times to make sure that oxygen is being bound and carbon dioxide is being released. Mind you, this process is taking place every second -- on average 20-30,000 times a day. It is something we simply take for granted.

The Purpose of the Skin

The skin, although very thin, is the largest organ of the body. It is designed to protect the body as well as excrete toxins from the body. There are three primary areas by which the body excretes toxins via sweat. It is through the armpits, the groin area, and behind the knee.

This system also allows for regulation of temperature to take place via the blood supply to the superficial aspect of the tissue. Toxins are released through the skin when there is opportunity to do so. By using too many products on our skin, we are interfering with our natural ability to release toxins from the body.

The skin is an amazing system. As the largest organ, it comprises 16% of our body weight. The skin serves many functions. It is designed to protect us from infections due to injury. It serves as a protective coating from the effects of ultraviolet light through the production of melanin which it produces upon exposure to sun. Vitamin D3, the precursor to Vitamin D, which is essential for the formation of healthy bones, is found in melanin.

Skin also acts as a temperature regulator during hot and cold conditions. It does this through a staggering supply of blood that runs along the superficial layer of the skin. In fact, in hot climates blood flow to the skin can be as much as 7 times higher as is normal, while during cold conditions blood flow is almost undetectable. This system allows the transference of heat to the surface when it is needed to remove heat from the body.

The skin also acts as a protective border. It is in a sense part of the immune system, able to identify foreign invaders and then stimulating the body's ability to protect itself from its environment. The skin also allows us to communicate with the world through its extraordinary sense of touch and feel.

The Liver

The liver is located along the lower right aspect of the abdomen. What is so important about the liver? You see, the liver has many functions in the body. Among them is its role in the absorption of fats and fat-soluble vitamins. The liver also stores and releases energy as it controls blood sugar. It regulates fat storage, aids in digestion through the production of bile, and regulates blood clotting. It produces hormones in our body and filters blood which helps protect the body from harmful substances as blood flows into the liver via the stomach and intestines. This is important especially if we are removing bacteria and poisons that we are exposed to in our daily lives.

The liver also creates cholesterol, which is necessary to every cell in the body. It produces Vitamin D, and stores minerals such as iron. Again this is all done without your awareness of it. It doesn't take a break; like the heart, brain, and lungs, the liver works all the time.

The Kidneys

Each of us is born with two kidneys. They are located just below the rib cage. Each kidney has millions of tiny tubules called nephrons. These nephrons are designed to filter the blood that circulates through it.

The kidney reabsorbs important substances that are needed for normal function in the body. The main functions of the kidneys are to filter waste from the body and retain substances that are needed such as proteins, glucose, minerals, and water. As this is all done, the kidney is able to maintain electrolyte balance.

Kidneys are important for the production of Vitamin D, which is needed for the maintenance of healthy bones. It also produces hormones which regulate blood pressure, as well as producing the hormone designed to make red blood cells. These are just some of the things that your kidneys do for you, every day, without you having to think about it.

The Eyes

The human eyeball is a sphere approximately 4 centimeters in size. There are millions of cells that allow for the amazing feat of vision to take place. This being said, scan the room, and take a look at what you see. Try to really absorb it all. As you do this you will begin to realize that you are using a sense called sight.

Sight has an amazing spectrum to it. It is able to see millions of shades of color. This perceptual system is designed to allow different shades of color and light and different shapes all to be absorbed and understood almost instantly. The eyes can see about 3 billion colors. This is almost impossible to comprehend, especially when we are so conditioned to identify colors as simply red, blue, green, yellow, black, and white.

The Hands

There are 13 different muscles in the hand. There are also 27 different bones. This allows for an incredible level of precision when picking up objects, playing the most difficult piano pieces, painting a portrait, or playing sports. All of these feats require a tremendous level of skill, yet we rarely think about what movements our hands are making as we do them. We are usually just concentrating on the task to be accomplished by our hands.

The Ears

Our hearing is an amazing creation allowing us to hear the most beautiful songs, the most cherished sounds of the ocean, the voices of our parents, children, and other loved ones. We are able to hear something that can change our life forever using these two little organs in our body called the ears.

The Muscles

There are 650 muscles within the human body. A staggering 650! They are designed to propel us forward and allow us to maintain our balance in relation to gravity. They protect our internal organs, as well as provide a tremendous level of strength. This again is done without our conscious effort.

We may realize the magnitude of the work the muscles do when we need to exert extra strength. However, there are so many functions of the muscles we take for granted. When was the last time you consciously thought about raising your arm up to reach for something or scratch your head?

The Skeletal System

The skeletal system is made up of 206 bones. These bones are designed to protect our internal organs and to provide resiliency against forces. They allow us to walk upright. There are many functions for the skeletal system not the least of which is the formation of red blood cells in the bone marrow. We will be talking in great detail about the utter importance that the skeletal system has on your overall well being as it relates to chiropractic. You will be very surprised indeed on the true impact that it has on all of us.

Complex movements are achieved within the skeletal system, and yet it is capable of functioning for 80-100 years without a problem. There is a great deal you can do through nutrition and exercise that is necessary to maintain the skeletal system. This is important in order to minimize any harmful deterioration which can take place at any age if you fail to properly maintain the skeletal system.

Chapter 5

The Health Model vs the Sick Model

One important and positive way that health care is changing is that it's moving from a "sick care" model to a "well care" model. What does this mean? Well, in years past, most health care was provided on a reactive basis, meaning that you only went to the doctor when you are sick. Today, healthcare is moving toward a "well care" model, in which a proactive approach is taken instead, through an ongoing relationship with a primary care practitioner (PCP).

The Health Model (also known as the 'wellness model') is a theory in caring for clients and patients that take the focus from being sick to preventative care. In the wellness model, there is a strong emphasis on holistic care where the client or patient is encouraged to take part in healthy activities that create a stronger body and mind that can ward off illness, instead of relying on the traditional health system to care for a sick body. Wellness is not just a set of practices that are incorporated at the doctor's office, but rather it's a change in lifestyle. Wellness includes care from your regular physician but also can include chiropractic, massage, nutrition, fitness and mental health care. All of these things make you a healthier person.

Health Care vs. Sick Care

Health care is wellness. It's everything that helps you move towards health and prevent problems from occurring again or even in the first place. This includes things like nutrition, exercise, whole food supplements, dental care, chiropractic care, massage, and acupuncture.

Think of it this way. Imagine a spectrum. Health is on one end of the spectrum, and sickness is on the other end of the spectrum. Your position on this spectrum can shift toward one side or the other depending on several factors. On the health end of the spectrum, the focus is on prevention and being proactive in doing things to promote and support health. On the sick end, the focus is on addressing the crisis and being reactive to the disease or illness.

Sick care is, in essence, damage control. The obvious need for "sick care" is in emergency situations, such as accidents, traumas, and other life-or-death acute conditions. Management of chronic conditions like heart disease, cancer, and diabetes is also included in "sick care." The main goal of "sick care" is to stop you from getting worse. The secondary goal is to make you feel better but not necessarily correct the cause of your problem. The "sick care" model rarely focuses on moving you back towards health and preventing the problem from occurring again.

The Wellness Approach

Wellness care seeks to turn on the natural healing ability, not by adding something to the system, but by removing anything that might interfere with normal function and trusting the body to know what to do if nothing were interfering with it. Standard medical care, on the other hand, seeks to treat a symptom by adding something from the outside - a medication, a surgery or procedure.

Wellness is a state of optimal conditions for normal function. The wellness approach is to look for underlying causes of any disturbance or disruption (which may or may not be causing symptoms at the time) and make changes in lifestyle that would optimize the conditions for normal function. That environment encourages natural healing, and minimizes the need for invasive treatment, which, in theory, should be administered only when absolutely necessary. When the body is working properly, it tends to heal effectively, no matter what the condition. This is true for mental and emotional health as well as physical health. While some people may suffer psychological disorders, creating an atmosphere of mental and emotional wellness will address all but the most serious problems.

Preventative Healthcare

Health is a state of wholeness in which your body knows its ever-changing needs and responds to those, all on its own. I believe that chiropractic care is a long-term form of preventative healthcare that maintains your body's nervous system to keep you in good health for a lifetime.

Chiropractic care doesn't heal injuries; rather, it helps the body to engage its own incredible natural healing abilities through a long-term routine of preventative healthcare maintenance for the nervous system.

Preventative healthcare through chiropractic focuses on your entire nervous system: your brain, spinal cord, and every one of the millions of nerve connections throughout your body. It monitors your entire body and all its needs, to help control and coordinate the necessary responses that allow the body to learn, adapt and constantly maintain its own health and wellness.

Preventative Care vs. Sick Care

The common healthcare model in the United States is the sick care model. It only looks at your body after symptoms of illness present, and then considers how best to treat these symptoms.

The preventative healthcare chiropractic model, on the other hand, is entirely natural, non-invasive, doesn't rely on chemicals, and looks to the root cause of your underlying health issues. It is focused entirely on correcting spinal subluxations to allow your whole nervous system to communicate better and increase the body's overall healing abilities. This improves your ability to adapt to stress and a variety of health conditions and helps to restore you to normal, healthy and optimal function. Chiropractic can restore your natural healing capability, and provide increased vitality, energy, bodily functions and overall health.

Hospitals and the Wellness Sham

Furthermore, while hospitals and health systems may preach wellness, few offer comprehensive services designed to improve your health and well-being. Rather, they pay lip-service to this essential component of health care – viewing wellness more as a marketing opportunity than a true effort to do everything in their power to minimize unnecessary and costly utilization of their medical services.

There's really no surprise here. Afterall, a healthy person does not make a good customer!

How to Move from Sickness to Wellness

Making the change from the sickness model to the wellness model can be a big challenge for some of our clients. The reality is, moving from a sickness state of mind to a wellness state of mind is incredibly personal. It is possible to shift from a sick-care system that doles out interventions to manage the burden of chronic illness to a positive health system, focused on wellness/well-being system that minimizes unnecessary utilization by focusing on population health. However, it would require tremendous will on the part of the people to achieve such a powerful transformation.

The key to transitioning from one model to the other is time, will power, and support. When we meet a new client who can benefit from the wellness model, we address their immediate issues, and then create a positive and encouraging atmosphere that they can feel comfortable expanding into. If they've come to see us for chiropractic care, we may encourage them to support that function with a visit a massage therapist or a fitness trainer. Treating the whole body with kindness and mindfulness is often all it takes to move a client from being "sick" to being "well."

Our Role In Changing The System

Now the question becomes whether we have the fortitude to change the healthcare paradigm, as well as accept the personal responsibility for our health that is essential to success. Below are the roles for each of us to play:

Government: There needs to be dramatically increased spending on proven prevention programs that can be administered at a local, state, or federal level. Furthermore, there need to be greater rewards under governmental reimbursement programs for those providers who embrace risk and demonstrate their ability to reduce the morbidity of a defined population.

Consumers/Patients: We need to understand what it means to be prudent stewards of our health, and the health of our families. It is essential that we understand the role lifestyle choices make in determining our health, and how we might combat risk-factors that impactl our future. For many of us, we will need to have access to resources that will aid in this journey – particularly if we are socio-economically challenged, and thus find lifestyle change all the more difficult.

Providers: Healthcare providers need to take the moral high-ground and do the right things for the communities they serve. One place to begin is with the development of a strategic wellness plan illustrating how wellness initiatives can be integrated into the very fabric of your hospital or health system's care model. Once developed and implemented, you can then reasonably assert that you do everything possible to minimize unnecessary consumption of health care resources while maximizing the health and well-being of your patients.

Insurers/Payers: There needs to be an unremitting pressure to partner more fully with providers on the assumption of risk for the health and well-being of a defined population, thus accelerating the demise of fee-for-service medicine, and its replacement with a reimbursement mechanism that rewards wellness.

Employers: There needs to be broader adoption and implementation of wellness programs that incorporate proven mechanisms for elevating the health and well-being of an employed population. Such programs will likely involve potent incentives for lifestyle modification by those employees at risk.

It's time to put the "health" back in healthcare. Physicians must join with other health care practitioners whose focus is on building health and wellness and not just managing disease and illness. Drugs and surgeries target the main complaint and symptoms but they fail to address the cause of the problems plaguing their patients. No amount of medication will address the true cause of degenerative diseases if the dysfunction within the body is not identified and restored. The irony is that the majority of the top 10 causes of death in modern society are rooted in diet and lifestyle (heart disease, certain cancers, diabetes, Alzheimer's – to name a few). These conditions may never have grown to their current epic proportions if the medical community would have continued to honor the fundamental health building values of diet and exercise.

Chapter 6

Where does United States (Western Medicine) Rank in Life Expectancy?

Until the early 1990s, despite the accomplishments of certain high-income countries in achieving significant continued improvements in life expectancy at birth, there was considerable disagreement among gerontologists and demographers as to what the future might bring. On the one hand, pessimists believed that the deaths above age 80 were due to problems associated with senescence and intractable aging processes. Consequently, increases in longevity beyond age 85 or so were unlikely to be achievable without fundamental biomedical breakthroughs that would affect those processes themselves. On the other hand, optimists believed that continued improvements in life expectancy were to be expected and that the official population projections of the time were too conservative.

We've known for years that Americans tend to be overweight and sedentary and that our health care system, despite being the most expensive in the world, produces some less-than-stellar results. People who closely follow the news may even have known that we live shorter lives than people in other wealthy nations and that infants in the U.S. die from various causes at far higher rates.

The report was prepared by a panel of doctors, epidemiologists, demographers, and other researchers charged by the National Research Council and the Institute of Medicine to better understand Americans' comparative health. They examined when and why people die in the U.S. and 16 other countries, including Australia, Japan, Canada, and nations in Western Europe. The data they pulled -- from such bodies as the World Health Organization and the Organization for Economic Cooperation and Development -- already existed, but no one had yet examined it this comprehensively.

The results surprised even the researchers. To their alarm, they said, they found a "strikingly consistent and pervasive" pattern of poorer health at all stages of life, from infancy to childhood to adolescence to young adulthood to middle and old age. Compared to people in other developed nations, Americans die far more often from injuries and homicides. We suffer more deaths from alcohol and other drugs and endure some of the worst rates of heart disease, lung disease, obesity, and diabetes.

These disproportionate deaths primarily affect young people. For three decades, Americans, particularly men, have had either the lowest or near the lowest likelihood of surviving to age 50. The most powerful reasons found for that were homicide, car accidents, other kinds of accidents, non-communicable diseases, and perinatal problems like low birth weight and premature birth, which contribute to high infant mortality.

Among the most striking of the report's findings are that among the countries studied, the U.S. has:

- The highest rate of death by violence, by a stunning margin
- The highest rate of death by car accident, also dramatically so
- The highest chance that a child will die before age 5
- The second-highest rate of death by coronary heart disease
- The second-highest rate of death by lung disease
- The highest teen pregnancy rate
- The highest rate of women dying due to complications of pregnancy and childbirth

The report does reveal bright spots: Americans are more likely to survive cancer or stroke, and if we live to age 75 we're likely to keep on living longer than others. But these advances are dwarfed by the grave shortcomings.

Where Does U.S. Rank In Crisis Care Intervention?

The World Health Report 2000, Health Systems: Improving Performance, ranked the U.S. health care system 37th in the world— a result that has frequently been discussed during the current debate on U.S. health care reform.

Despite having the most expensive health care system, the United States ranks last overall among 11 industrialized countries on measures of health system quality, efficiency, access to care, equity, and healthy lives, according to a Commonwealth Fund report. The other countries included in the study were Australia, Canada, France, Germany, the Netherlands, New Zealand, Norway, Sweden Switzerland, and the United Kingdom. While there is room for improvement in every country, the U.S. stands out for having the highest costs and lowest performance—the U.S. spent $8,508 per person on health care in 2011, compared with $3,406 in the United Kingdom, which ranked first overall.

Despite the claim by many in the U.S. health policy community that international comparison is not useful because of the uniqueness of the United States, the rankings have figured prominently in many areas. It is hard to ignore that in 2006, the United States was number 1 in terms of health care spending per capita but ranked 39th for infant mortality, 43rd for adult female mortality, 42nd for adult male mortality, and 36th for life expectancy. These facts have fueled a question now being discussed in academic circles, as well as by government and the public: Why do we spend so much to get so little?

The current proposals for U.S. health care reform focus mostly on extending insurance coverage, decreasing the growth of costs through improved efficiency, and expanding prevention and wellness programs. The policy debate has been overwhelmingly centered on the first two of these elements. Achieving universal insurance coverage in the United States would protect households against undue financial burdens at the same time that it was saving an estimated 18,000 to 44,000 lives. However, narrowing the gap in health outcomes between the United States and other high-income countries or even slowing its descent in the rankings would require much more than insurance expansion.

Why Does Western Medicine Insist On Using Crisis Care Tactics For Prevention Situations?

Although we talk about a "health care" system and health care reform, what we're actually talking about is a "disease care" system and disease care reform. Doctors of modern western medicine are trained to treat disease with drugs and surgery. They are not trained to keep people healthy.

At medical school, the doctors are taught how to treat the symptoms of the disease, rather than how to prevent disease in the first place. For example, throughout the training, they receive very few lectures on nutrition, despite the fact that diet is fundamental to good health. Nor are they trained in other lifestyle modalities that help keep people well, such as exercise and relaxation therapies. They are taught nothing about the wisdom of alternative medical systems that have been helping other cultures for centuries.

I will be the first to acknowledge that modern western medicine and science have made phenomenal advances. These improvements alleviate pain and suffering and save lives every day. Better treatment of trauma and burns for example, or the management of acute medical and surgical emergencies, are among the miracles of modern life. We have drugs today that, when used appropriately, work wonders. We are indeed blessed to have modern western medicine in our arsenal, and for disasters like the Haiti earthquake, this kind of medicine is life-saving.

In a true health care system, we must use modern western medicine for what it is good at - crisis care, acute medical and surgical emergencies - and natural, non-toxic and non-invasive therapies whenever possible. The most effective ways of preventing and treating most chronic diseases are diet, supplements, exercise, stress management and other benign modalities. And herein lies the rub. Although guidance may be helpful, lifestyle changes can't be imposed from above - they have to come from you. There is no greater reward than being the master of your health.

When Did Insurance Companies Come About?

The history of insurance consisted of the development of the modern business of insurance against risks, especially regarding cargo, property, death, automobile accidents, and medical treatment. The industry helps to eliminate risks (as when fire insurance companies demand the implementation of safe practices and the installation of hydrants), spreads risks from the individual to the broader community, and provides an important source of long-term finance for both the public and private sectors. The insurance industry is profitable and provides attractive employment opportunities for white-collar workers.

In the United States, health insurance is any program that helps pay for medical expenses, whether through privately purchased insurance, social insurance or a social welfare program funded by the government. Synonyms for this usage include "health coverage," "health care coverage" and "health benefits." In a more technical sense, the term is used to describe any form of insurance that protects against the costs of medical services. This usage includes private insurance and social insurance programs, such as Medicare, which pools resources and spreads the financial risk associated with major medical expenses across the entire population to protect everyone, as well as social welfare programs such as Medicaid and the Children's Health Insurance Program which assist people who cannot afford health coverage.

In addition to medical expense insurance, "health insurance" may also refer to insurance covering disability or long-term nursing or custodial care needs. Different health insurance provides different levels of financial protection, and the scope of coverage can vary widely, with more than 40 percent of insured individuals reporting that their plans do not adequately meet their needs as of 2007.

Today, the internet has changed the insurance industry by blowing the field wide open. Now people can go online to find the cheapest rate, even as companies shop internationally for the right coverage. This is one source of motivation for companies to merge with other financial services. The increase in size gives them a global market and the integration of services gives them a domestic advantage with customers who are more concerned with convenience than price.

When Were The First Hospitals Created?

Pennsylvania Hospital happens to be the first hospital created. It is was founded in 1751 by Dr. Thomas Bond and Benjamin Franklin "to care for the sick-poor and insane who were wandering the streets of Philadelphia." At the time, Philadelphia was the fastest growing city in the 13 colonies. In 1730, the population numbered 11,500 and had grown to 15,000 by 1750 (the city continued to grow, and by 1776, its 40,000 residents made Philadelphia the second largest English-speaking city in the British Empire).

At the time, colonial America's urban centers were far healthier than their European counterparts. Nevertheless, the Philadelphia region, according to city leaders of the day, was "a melting pot for diseases, where Europeans, Africans, and Indians engaged in a free exchange of their respective infections." Faced with increasing numbers of the poor who were suffering from physical illness and the increasing numbers of people from all classes suffering from mental illness, civic-minded leaders sought a partial solution to the problem by founding a hospital.

The idea for the hospital originated with Dr. Thomas Bond. Born in Calvert County, Maryland, Bond, a Quaker, moved to Philadelphia as a young man. In 1738, to further his medical education, he went abroad to study medicine in London. While in Europe, Bond spent time at the famous French hospital, the Hotel-Dieu in Paris, and became impressed with the continent's new hospital movement. Bond returned to Philadelphia in 1739 and two years later was appointed Port Inspector for Contagious Diseases.

When Did Medical Doctors Go From Private Practices and Into Hospital Groups?

There is a dangerous trend underway in American healthcare: The death of the private practice doctor's office. This is a deliberate trend driven primarily by federal policymakers, and it does not bode well for either the cost of healthcare or the health of individual patients.

Hospitals justified their mergers by claiming they helped reach economies of scale. But the mergers also reduced competition, helping the hospital systems negotiate higher reimbursements from health insurers.Then came the A.C.A., which envisioned large, integrated provider networks, and the government was willing to hand out billions of dollars to providers that successfully implemented the government's vision of quality care.The effects on physicians and patients are unclear. But in a government-run health care chess game, both are just pawns.

The small, independent medical practices have long dominated the medical landscape. But increasingly, doctors are giving up their independence to join larger groups or hospital systems, often getting help with back-office functions like billing and insurance negotiations while staying in their old offices and seeing the same patients.

The idea is that by teaming up, doctors and hospitals can avoid repeat tests and offer the best possible care at the lowest price. It's a notion that has long been percolating in the healthcare field. They're sensing that change is necessary, and they want and desire and need perhaps a partnership with a health system. So our timetable to get there into accountable care and truly clinically integrated system have sped up.

Choosing between private practice and working at a hospital may be a weighty decision for doctors, but patients may not notice much of a difference.

When did the sub specialization of medicine begin.and when did it become so compartmentalized?

The recent decline in the production of primary care physicians has been associated with a decrease in the production of general internists and an increase in the number of medical subspecialists. A significant majority of entering internal medicine residents anticipate entering a medical subspecialty. This transition in the development of the medical workforce, perceived by some as inappropriate, is analyzed in light of historical trends in the evolution of internal medicine and its subspecialties, and in conjunction with the roles played by the American Board of Internal Medicine and the National Institutes of Health. The evidence is presented that the creation of virtually independent subspecialty departments may have been detrimental to the education of physicians and not productive of the physician-scientists they are assumed to create.

As medical scientists specialized and devoted their intellectual energies to understanding more and more about narrower topic areas, general practitioners differentiated into physicians with specific areas of expertise, devoting some or all of their work to that specific area. The first medical specialty to create its assessment board was ophthalmology in 1917. Prompted by the growth of optometry as a separate discipline, the American Medical Association and the American Ophthalmological Society established an independent board of specialists to create standards that would recognize physicians whose knowledge and skills demonstrated expertise in identifying and treating disorders of the eye.

Also, the new specialties can benefit both patients and physicians. However, a proliferation of specialties without adequate justification may simply confuse the public without creating a social good. The use of specified criteria can lead to rational decision-making that balances the potential benefit of recognizing more specific expertise to the detriment of fragmentation of the profession. This approach extends beyond traditional specialization, which requires formal training, to the recognition of new areas of expertise that physicians gain while in practice — that is, focused practice.

What About Medicare and Medicaid and How They Are Funded?

Medicare is an entitlement program that provides health insurance to persons aged 65 and older or to those with disabilities without regard to income. Medicaid is health insurance available to certain people and families who have limited income and resources. It covers an estimated 58 million people. Medicaid is overseen by the federal government, but each state establishes its eligibility standards and determines the scope of services. States also set the rate of payment for services, and administer their own Medicaid programs.

Like Medicare, Medicaid is overseen by the Centers for Medicare and Medicaid Services of the Department of HHS.

The Medicare program, enacted in 1965, provides seniors with health insurance coverage comparable to that available to non-elderly and non-disabled Americans in the private sector. It includes hospital insurance (Part A), supplementary insurance (Part B) to cover outpatient and home health services as well as physician visits, and prescription drug coverage (Part D). Seniors also have the choice to enroll in private plans (Part C), called Medicare Advantage, to cover their services. The Medicare program covers 44 million people, 37 million seniors, and 7 million disabled Americans. It is funded by Federal payroll taxes, general tax revenues, and beneficiary premiums. Medicare is administered by the Centers for Medicare & Medicaid Services (CMS).

The Medicaid program is jointly funded by the federal government and states. The federal government pays states for a specified percentage of program expenditures, called the Federal Medical Assistance Percentage (FMAP). States must ensure they can fund their share of Medicaid expenditures for the care and services available under their state plan.

States can establish their own Medicaid provider payment rates within federal requirements, and pay for services through fee-for-service or managed care arrangements. To change the way they pay Medicaid providers, states must submit a State Plan Amendment (SPA) for CMS review and approval.

Why Can't We Buy Health Insurance like Auto Insurance?

During the debate over health insurance reform, you'll occasionally run into the idea that health insurance should be provided more like auto insurance. After all, in most states, everyone has to have auto insurance, so everyone's covered. If you have a decent driving record, you'll have lots of choices among providers; and most people can find the minimum required insurance, even if it's in a high-risk pool.

If the market works for auto insurance, why not health insurance? The answer is simple: People and cars are different. We (rightly) value them differently. And the market can't account for that difference. Here's why:

First, car insurance is a very restrictive form of catastrophic coverage. It doesn't cover the everyday items that keep cars running, like oil changes; nor does it cover mechanical breakdowns, even when they cost you a fortune. You can put off an oil change, and eventually, your car will break down, but your auto insurance won't help you then. It only comes into play when you hit someone/something, or they/it hit you.

Your health is different. Your body can break down in numerous ways – cancer, pneumonia, or a collision with a bus, for example. To be effective, health insurance has to cover both preventative and catastrophic care, because the two are inextricably connected. People will put off a yearly check-up if insurance doesn't cover it. And when small health problems go unnoticed or untreated, they become full-blown problems that cost a great deal more to treat in an emergency room.

Health insurance reform is about ensuring everyone has more than catastrophic coverage or the emergency room to rely on — because it's healthier and cheaper for everyone, and ultimately better for our communities and our economy. If everyone can easily access and afford preventative care, that means fewer expensive trips to the emergency room.

A better analogy for health insurance is the local fire or police department. It doesn't matter how much you earn, or how high up the social ladder you are; you get the same fire engine. Maybe you can afford better home monitoring and security if you are wealthy, but you don't get better fire engines or faster patrol cars. And you don't get a bill in the mail when a fire is put out, or a burglar is caught.

Chapter 7

What Is Going on With

The Opioid Epidemic in The United States?

Almost 100,000 people died in the United States last year because of drug overdoses, according to reports from National Public Radio. This staggering number means that nearly a million people have died from a drug overdose since the beginning of the opioid crisis that still grips the US that started back in the late nineties. In 2019, opioids are involved in over 70% of drug overdose deaths according to the CDC. To fully understand this crisis and the repercussions of it, you need to understand how it started.

What Are Opioid Painkillers and How Are They Used?

Opioids are narcotic drugs derived from opium poppy, like heroin. Opioid painkillers are painkillers also derived from opium poppy or made synthetically to have the same type of effects as opioids, like the often deadly fentanyl, and some other pain relievers that are only available by prescription. Aside from very acute injuries and patients in hospice care, most of these drugs should not be used outside of a hospital setting. The remaining narcotic pain medications classified as opioids, such as morphine, oxycodone (often known by its brand name OxyContin®) and hydrocodone (often known by its brand name Vicodin®) may be prescribed for use to relieve acute pain for very short periods of time, and even in these cases the drugs still pose a risk to the patients who use them.

Opioid pain relievers were found to be effective for use as breakthrough pain relievers for cancer patients. Then began the slippery slope of doctors prescribing these types of painkillers for patients with *any* type of chronic pain. The difference in dealing with chronic pain is that chronic pain is long term and opioid pain relievers are not a long term answer. In fact, for an otherwise healthy person expecting to live a long life, these types of painkillers are the absolute wrong answer.

Why Opioid Pain Relievers Do Not Work for Chronic Pain

When a patient is dealing with chronic pain, the top priority should be to stop the pain by stopping what is causing it. Pain is like your body's alarm system. In this way, prescribing pain pills for chronic pain is like shutting off a fire alarm, but not attempting to put out the fire!

Beyond the obvious problem of simply masking pain while other problems continue and therefore may continue to damage the body, opioid pain relievers are addictive. These types of painkillers also become tolerated by the body so that the patient will need stronger and stronger doses to achieve the same effects. Should a person in this condition then have an accidental acute injury, there is simply no medicine that will be effective as pain relief for them.

Furthermore, opioid pain relievers in and of themselves damage the body. Long term use can damage many different bodily systems including the respiratory, central nervous, gastrointestinal, cardiovascular, immune, musculoskeletal, and endocrine systems.

Why Opioid Pain Relievers Do Not Work for Injuries

While it is normal for a doctor to give a patient a narcotic pain medication in the immediate aftermath of an injury to help handle the initial pain of resetting a bone or recovering from a surgery, this type of medicine should be discontinued immediately once the initial stage has passed. This is very important because if you are in extraordinary pain beyond this point, something is wrong and you will need to make sure that it is corrected.

After most surgeries and bad injuries you will see a physical therapist, chiropractor and other types of medical professionals who can help you with rehabilitation and pain management. If you mask your pain, the medical professionals who are helping you will not be able to adequately assess your progress which can lead to problems that can keep you from healing correctly or even cause reinjury!

Opioid Addiction is More Insidious than Other Type of Addiction

Substance abuse is a prevalent problem in the US and other developed countries. Over the years much has been done to address this problem and educate the public about the dangers of drug abuse and substance addiction. The problem with opioid addiction is that it can be far more insidious than other types of drug addiction. This is because many people are completely unaware of the dangers of prescription pain relievers.

Many people are simply uneducated or even worse, misinformed about the dangers of narcotic pain medications. Here are just a few of the myths people believe about opioid pain relievers:

Myth #1

It's not dangerous if my doctor prescribed it.

False.

It doesn't matter where you obtain opioid painkillers, they are still dangerous, have terrible side effects, and are highly addictive.

Myth #2

Opioid painkillers are only addictive if you take them when you don't need them.

False.

One common mistake people make is to assume that because they are truly in need of pain relief that narcotic painkillers are not addictive. This is simply untrue. Whether you are in pain or not, opioid painkillers are still drugs with the exact same addictive properties either way. If you take them, you are putting yourself at risk for addiction.

Myth #3

If I am in pain, I should be prescribed pain medication.

False.

If you are in pain you have every right to seek pain relief, but narcotic pain medication should never be a first choice.

Sadly, these false beliefs lead people right into the throes of addiction. A person who would never directly make the decision to use illicit street drugs like heroin will gladly accept a prescription for hydrocodone from their doctor to stop a common pain such as low back pain. When this person tries to stop taking the drug, the pain will come back. Eventually they will need an even stronger pain killer to get relief. By the time anyone realizes there is an issue it is too late and the patient is now addicted. If the doctor realizes there is a problem and cuts off the supply, the patient may, out of desperation, seek the drug through less scrupulous means such as lying about their condition or even buying the drug illegally. This is how a legal prescription can easily turn into a substance abuse and even addiction problem.

How Bad is America's Opioid Epidemic Now?

At least 44 people die every day in the US as a result of a prescription opioid overdose, says the Center for Disease Control and Prevention. They confirm that drug overdose was also the leading cause of deaths caused by injury in the US in 2013 and among people 25 to 64 years of age, it caused more deaths than traffic accidents. These are absolutely terrifying statistics and the numbers continue to get worse every single year!

The CDC has urged doctors to prescribe fewer opioid prescriptions, pointing out that the increase in these prescriptions has helped to fuel the number of opioid related overdoses and deaths. According to the Department of Health and Human Services, one out of every three people who have prescription drug coverage through Medicare received at least one prescription for an opioid painkiller in 2016.

The problem has gotten so out of hand that both federal and state government officials have weighed in on the problem. The U.S. Government is doing all it can to curb the epidemic of prescription drug abuse, including enacting new legislation.

This wave of opioid deaths has culminated in the deadliest drug crisis in US history. Overdoses fueled by opioids are now the leading cause of death for Americans under 50 years of age, having killed more than 60,000 people just last year, which is more than guns, car accidents, or the H.I.V. epidemic at its peak.

To make matters even worse, these prescription opioid painkillers are proven to be a gateway for later use of heroin. So it is no surprise that use of that drug is now also on the rise. Heroin has devastated the US in recent years. The CDC reports that heroin use among young adults aged 18 to 25 has doubled in the past decade. With the increased use of the drug, heroin-related overdose deaths have also grown significantly, witnessing a four-fold increase since 2010 and that trend seems to be continuing.

What is Driving America's Opioid Epidemic?

In recent decades, the incidents of chronic pain have dramatically increased at the same time healthcare costs have skyrocketed. This came at a time when doctors were becoming even more aware of patients' need for pain control as well as patient advocacy groups lobbying for better pain management. Couple this with weak pharmaceutical oversight and a deceptive and illegal push from drug makers to prescribe more of their specific drugs (Purdue Pharma, maker of OxyContin and other opioid drugs admitted their guilt in a 2020 court case) and you can see how the situation set the stage for a substance abuse crisis.

Now, the US is faced with name brand OxyContin being the most popular recreational drug among high school seniors. Furthermore, it is popular among the stars of Hollywood and music, many of which have even admitted to using it. The opioid epidemic has gone well beyond a simple matter of over prescribing. All forms of opioid painkillers have not just permeated, but rather saturated the black market. They have acted as a gateway drug leading thousands to use illicit street drugs, and many to even die from an overdose of drugs like heroin and fentanyl.

At the end of the day, a perfect storm of monetary greed and medical negligence has led the US down this road. While greed is easy to understand, medical negligence is not. To understand how and why doctors were complicit in this situation, you have to consider that many doctors in the US are actually in a very delicate position. Most doctors are not paid by their patients and do not therefore feel as responsible to their patients as they may have years ago. Doctors are paid by insurance companies, the government, and unfortunately, many times, by pharmaceutical companies in the form of bonuses, gifts, and perks. Doctors often times act more responsible to these entities before they are to their patients. Beyond that, many American doctors are overworked and cannot spend the time that they should be diagnosing and treating their patients. Pressure from insurance and pharmaceutical companies, added to pressure from patients in pain (some already badly addicted to narcotic pain killers) pushed many doctors to write prescriptions for opioid painkillers that they should not have written. Of course, there were also those who may write prescriptions for pure profit and the 2000's have seen plenty of those stripped of their licenses and even jailed in some cases.

Where Does the American Opioid Crisis Go from Here?

Aside from the obvious direct effects of the opioid crisis, there are many other indirect and unseen effects as well. The devastation created by the illegal drug trade which has been so fueled by opioids as of late, cannot even be measured. Opioid addiction has been at the root of more thefts, burglaries, robberies and murders because people become desperate to get their hands on more drugs and often times, this can lead to devastating consequences.

The US government, as well as American society, has begun to fight back. There are new laws about how and when these extremely potent and dangerous drugs can be prescribed. There is oversight to ensure doctors are not over prescribing these drugs anymore. Further, the drug dealers who sell these types of drugs illegally, from prescription painkillers to fentanyl to heroin, are being pursued and prosecuted with far more vigor than in years past. They face much longer sentences as well.

Unfortunately, one place the US really lags behind is in treatment for addiction. Sadly as long as there are addicts willing to pay there will be someone willing to sell illegal drugs no matter how stiff the penalty is. This means that treating addiction will need to become a serious priority in the US, and will likely cost billions of dollars. As it stands there are far too few treatment facilities for those with addiction and substance abuse problems and generally speaking substance abuse problems do not leave most people with extra funds to spend on treatment once they have hit rock bottom.

How Can the Opioid Crisis Be Stopped?

There is no quick and easy answer to this question. Obviously the efforts in place will need to be continued and they will likely even need to be stepped up. Having the general public better educated on matters pertaining to opioid addiction is a great place to start. The US will need to invest in more and better policing of these drugs. Even stiffer penalties for selling opioids may need to be enacted. Certainly, there will need to be more facilities and professionals dedicated to the treatment of substance abuse and addiction to be able to help those who are afflicted.

These are the methods that we can use to clean up the problem, but it doesn't really get at the core issue. The core issue is that too many people were desperately left in pain for many years and medical doctors either failed to treat the pain or chose to mask it with drugs. This has left many patients who experience chronic pain skeptical about going to the hospital or taking any kind of prescriptions.

What is needed now for patients who must recover from injuries or surgery or who have chronic pain, is a better way to handle pain. Now is the time to begin to use effective methods of pain control that are not addictive, do not cause side effects, and hopefully involve far less surgeries and procedures.

Better Pain Management

Patients should never have to unnecessary suffer from pain. However, treating the symptom of pain and not treating the root cause of the pain is also unacceptable. Pain medication should only be given to a patient as a last and final resort when there are no other options available and the medication will do less harm than the pain will.

When it comes to current pain management techniques, alternative therapies (as they were once called) are no longer considered so alternative. With more time and study, many of these methods have been proven effective. Laser therapy, for example, has been proven in many studies to be effective for pain relief.

Laser therapy, sometimes called cold laser therapy, is great for relieving pain. The laser is used to reduce inflammation and stimulate the cells so that they repair themselves faster and more completely. Lasers have also been found to be very effective on chronic pain. Laser treatments are noninvasive and are not at all painful. Many people even enjoy their laser treatments!

Corrective exercises are another very effective way to control pain in many situations. You can learn these kinds of exercises from your physical therapist or chiropractor. These are not the calisthenics that you remember from gym class. These are exercises designed specifically to strengthen certain areas of the body. This can be used to either relieve pressure from another area or add extra support to an area to prevent future injuries.

Chiropractic care is also another great tool in the toolbox when it comes to pain management. It might seem a bit foreign if you have never had it done but people who have had chiropractic adjustments soften swear by it, and the science is there to back it up. The amazing thing about having a chiropractic adjustment is that because it effectively works to increase the flexibility and flow of the spine, it often works to treat the main cause of pain as well as relieving the pain itself.

Generally speaking, you will find that when it comes to pain relief your best options may be to see a chiropractor. Another advantage to seeing a chiropractor to help manage your pain as opposed to seeing a medical physician is that while medical physicians are often busy with many patients only spending a few minutes with each one, a chiropractor is much more hands on. Chiropractors work with you personally and tailor your treatments to meet your specific needs and help with your specific problems.

What You Can Do to Avoid Opioid Addiction

It is of the utmost importance that you remember that it is you and only you who should be making decisions about how to care for your body. Your medical doctors work for you; they are not an authority over you or your healthcare. As much as everyone wants to believe that their doctor is in their corner, it is also necessary to evaluate every situation yourself. As has been seen in the past, anyone can have ulterior motives in their actions. This isn't even always malevolent as it may well be subconscious or situational. For these reasons, take any doctor's recommendations very seriously, but make your own decisions.

You should never, ever, be afraid to turn down a prescription or ask for a second opinion. Ideally, you will want to have a good enough relationship with any professional that treats you that you will feel comfortable telling them how you feel about pain management and what you feel that your needs are. No doctor should ever pressure you to treat your pain in a way that you feel is inappropriate or irresponsible. Taking prescription pain medication should be an absolute last resort only when you know what is causing your pain and have already exhausted every other pain management option available.

More and more research validates how effective many non-drug related approaches are when it comes to relieving pain, especially chronic pain. Therapies such as acupuncture, laser therapy, massage therapy, physical therapy, chiropractic adjustments, meditation and yoga can have amazing effects on pain levels without the risk of addiction or side effects. Try these alternatives before you take a prescription painkiller.

Conclusion

The opioid crisis in the US has had devastating consequences across the board, from the loss of individual lives totaling in the hundreds of thousands, to the economic impact of the costs of drug rehabilitation to the deterioration of the fabric of our society as criminals commit robberies and murders to support the trade of this powerful drug.

While there are a few extreme situations that may call for narcotic painkillers, they generally should not be used outside of a hospital setting. Opioid painkillers are not only ineffective for treating chronic pain, but treating chronic pain with opioid painkillers will almost always lead to dependency, increased tolerance levels and addiction.

Some people mistakenly believe that opioid painkillers are not dangerous as long as they are prescribed, that they are not addictive if you are in pain and really need them or that pain pills are the only thing that will relieve pain. None of these things are true, and in fact, it is important to know that any time you take opioid painkillers there are risks. These types of painkillers are always addictive and their long term use will always result in damage to your body, no matter why you take them or whether or not they were prescribed.

America's opioid epidemic has only continued to grow and has gotten vastly worse over the last few decades. Spurred on by faulty and lazy legislation, poor enforcement, and extreme over prescribing, the opioid epidemic has affected so many people that almost everyone now knows someone who has been touched by it in some way. The epidemic has continued to be fueled by pharmaceutical companies and insurance companies pushing products and cheap fast results that do not last. As this epidemic of opioid drug abuse has continued to grow and ravage the country the federal and state governments have stepped in and attempted to help legislate a solution by regulating these types of drugs and severely prosecuting those who chose to sell them illegally. Measures like these will start to bring an end to the crisis, but the root of the problem still remains.

Better pain management, pain management without the use of damaging and dangerous drugs, has to be made available. Patients who deal with chronic pain need to be cared for with more thoughtfulness and insight into their individual situations and needs. Every other method should be exhausted before a doctor resorts to writing a prescription for a narcotic painkiller.

Patient education and responsibility is the key to ending the opioid crisis in the US. As a patient, you must take control of the situation and choose what is right for you. Avoid the use and therefore the risk of opioid pain medication. Opt to seek a second opinion, try an alternative therapy, or schedule an appointment with a chiropractor. Make sure that you as a patient make your health and wellbeing a priority over the big dollars of pharmaceutical companies. Remember that your treatment is your choice, and is in your hands. Make the best choice for your health and choose not to use opioid painkillers outside of a hospital setting.

Chapter 8

The Mistakes We Make Every Day

Each new day we make unconscious mistakes that are putting our spinal health and therefore, our overall wellness at stake. Some of the most common ones can be found here with ways to help improve upon or correct the mistakes.

There are simple adjustments we can make to improve posture and protect our necks and backs throughout the day. They show simple and subtle ways we can reduce tension that leads to trouble for our spine

Start the day off right with a good stretching session. Don't make the mistake of immediately jumping out of bed and getting in your car for a long car ride or right to your desk for work.

When brushing your teeth, don't hunch over the sink. Stand up straight and bend at the waist when you need to rinse.

Make sure chairs are the right height and depth for your body. Your feet should be flat on the floor, with your knees slightly slower than your hips. Your lower back should be well supported.

Ensure that you have adequate lighting for all tasks. One of the main causes of tension headaches is poor lighting and the eye strain that results. If you use the computer or electronic devices for a significant amount of time for your work, invest in some blue light filtering glasses. This is important for eye health as well as good sleep.

Avoid high-heeled shoes. They can cause spinal stress because the weight is not evenly distributed between heel and toe. It can also lead to foot and ankle problems in addition to back problems.

Sitting with your legs crossed in the same direction can eventually lead to spinal misalignment. Ideally you should sit with both feet on the floor.

Holding a cell phone with your shoulder can cause the spinal joints to lock up in the upper back, neck and shoulders. Use your hand or a headset if you need to have your hands free.

If you have a desk job, be sure to get up and move around frequently. It is important to change positions often, especially if while sitting you are doing repetitive motions, such as typing at a computer. It is also important to make sure your workstation is ergonomically set up correctly for you.

Find ways to reduce emotional stress and tension. That will carry into your posture if left to fester.

Get plenty of sleep on a quality mattress and good pillow that supports the neck and spine. We spend (or at least we should!) one third of our lives sleeping! Investing in a supportive mattress is a good investment!

Chapter 9

The Destructive Effects of Sugar

There is something that most of us consume daily that may be contributing to many of our health problems: SUGAR. Sadly, the average American consumes 2-3 pounds of sugar on a weekly basis. The number may seem exaggerated at first, but if we take into account that many types of sugars are sneakily "hidden" in multiple types of foods, such a high amount is not surprising at all. Processed sugar is often found in the form of white sugar (sucrose), corn syrup, and dextrose. These processed and concentrated kinds of sugar are often found in breakfast cereals, bread, jams, butters, condiments/sauces, peanut butter, pies, tomato sauce, and a broad range of processed and pre-made meals.

The average sugar intake in the U.S has risen from 25 pounds per individual a few decades ago to almost 135 pounds of sugar intake per person annually. Back in the 19th century, the average sugar intake per person was just 5 pounds annually. The levels of sugar intake keeps on rising at alarming rates with no indications of reversal. Another noteworthy observation is that up until the early 20th century, cancer and heart problem rates were almost non existent. Although there are probably many factors involve in our chronic disease epidemic currently, could our excess sugar intake be a contribution?

There has been some scientific evidence that demonstrates that the more sugar someone takes, the higher the risk of developing health problems later in their lives. From elevated cholesterol levels to lower immunity, sugar has a detrimental impact on our system.

Let's take a deeper dive into what sugar does to the body and how addictive it actually is.

The G.I (GLYCEMIC INDEX)

In order to acknowledge the mechanism of sugar within our system, we should be aware of the Glycemic Index (G.I) first. Every type of food that contains natural or synthetic sugar is measured according to its G.I. This index is used as a measure on a scale from 0 to 100 (the highest) in association with the impact of this sugar levels on blood glucose levels. Foods that are ranked with a low G.I are deemed to be more healthy and valuable for our bodies, while those with a high G.I score on the contrary, are considered to be unhealthy and damaging to our system as it will spike blood sugar levels.

Foods with a lower GI often are more beneficial to overall health because of the minimal effects they have on blood sugar. Here are just some of the health benefits if our diet consists more food lower on the GI:

- Decreased cholesterol levels

- Lower risk of developing Diabetes

- Increased energy levels

- Controlled cravings and hunger episodes

- Raises sensitivity to insulin

- More stable body weight and loss of excess fat

- Lower risk of developing heart diseases

It is important to be mindful of the GI when choosing your meals. Foods with a low G.I score release controlled amounts of sugar at more gradual speed in your system compared to foods with a high G.I score. The gradual release of sugar in the blood helps keep energy levels stabilized and prevents those infamous sudden sugar spikes which lead to energy crashes throughout the day. You will realize this happens to you and others, when you take high amounts of sugar after lunch time. If you took a high in sugar food during noon hours, you will most likely feel sleepy and ready to take a nap by 2 a.m.

The blood sugar levels raise to their peak about an hour after you eat a high sugary food, drink or high carb meal and then they fall suddenly after that hour passes. This is the culprit of energy crashes and tiredness after one hour or so of consuming something high in sugar. The "sugar crash" as we know it, is actually pretty common.

Link between Sugar and Cholesterol

Based on the findings of a University of Vermont study, there is connection between high blood lipid levels and sugar intake. The study further demonstrated that heightened consumption of sugar was also associated with elevated triglyceride levels and decreased levels of HDL (the beneficial) cholesterol. The research outcomes were so evident that the American Heart Association has also validated these findings in public.

The study had people taking raised amounts of sugar or high amounts of processed white sugar (sucrose). When these people took excess amounts of sugar, their triglyceride levels were heightened whereas their good HDL levels were quite low within their blood. Very low HDL levels are associated with a heightened risk of developing heart disease.

How is HDL cholesterol is beneficial for the system and why sugar has a destructive effect on our systems? You may already be aware that not all cholesterol/fat lipids are actually bad for your system. Having insufficient amounts of good HDL cholesterol can be very destructive to your heart and system. HDL is actually the beneficial cholesterol that circulates through the blood and carries mini lipoproteins that that act synergistically to cleanse the blood stream.

HDL performs the following beneficial functions in the system:

- HDL cleanses and strips from the bad lipids/LDL cholesterol through circulating small assistant lipo-proteins.

- HDL recycles bad cholesterol by sending it to the liver to be handed and reformed.

- HDL acts a maintenance group that repairs the internal linings of the blood vessels that became destructed through a procedure known as "atherosclerosis". HDL is the most ideal factor for cleansing the blood from bad cholesterol and keep the body functioning at its peak capacity. It actually unblocks the internal linings of blood vessels and prevents destruction coming from toughening of arterial walls (atherosclerosis), as stated earlier. Individuals who take high-sugary foods and drinks, smoke, are inactive, or are obese are more prone to develop heart disorders that those following healthier lifestyle habits. Overall, people with high levels of good HDL cholesterol are much less likely to develop heart problems whereas those with low HDL scores in their blood are more prone to develop heart disorders, among other health issues.

Sugar and Its Detrimental Impact on the Immune System

A study performed during the 1970s, demonstrated that a person's own white blood cells required amounts of Vitamin C to process and expel out of their system bacteria, viruses, and other intruders. White blood cells need 50X the amount of Vitamin C, to go through this phase within a cellular level. For the purpose of finding out how fast this procedure happens (also known as phagocytosis), a phagocytic index may be utilized. In the 70s, scientist Linus Pauling demonstrated through his trials that blood cells require adequate amounts of Vitamin C. He has found out that when someone has caught a cold, high amounts of Vitamin C are needed to treat cold/make it heal faster. Due to the fact that both Vitamin C and sugar have similar chemical forms, they antagonize each other when blood sugar levels get raised in the bloodstream. They two in reality rival each other to penetrate the cell. Therefore, when there are higher amounts of sugar present in the bloodstream, due to sugar intake, fewer amounts of Vitamin C to penetrate the cell. When we take high amounts of sugar, the immune system function will suffer as a result.

Up to this point, we have explained the common cold and how a rise in blood sugar levels hinders Vitamin C from penetrating the cell walls to fight the common cold virus but what happens in other disorders? The same principle is also applicable. Insulin struggles for its way to penetrate the cell when higher amounts of it are already existing within the cell than Vitamin C. This principle also applies to inflammatory disorders like diabetes, cancer, heart problems, and asthma. The common denominator here is the high intake of sugar.

Common sugars have been demonstrated to worsen health problems such as:

- Cancer
- Cardiovascular problems
- Arthritis
- Osteoporosis
- Diabetes
- Development of gallstones

Link between Cancer and Sugar

Regulating the provision of sugar in the bloodstream is very valuable for tackling cancer. There has been this old yet widespread notion that "cancer feeds on sugar". This has been proven to be accurate, but we need to understand better the mechanisms of such association.

In the early 1930s, German Scientist Otto Warburg, was awarded the Nobel prize for being the first to discover the energy metabolism of cancer cells as opposed to that of healthy cells. The final finding emerging from his trials was that cancer cells use sugar at a much more elevated pace than normal healthy cells. The more sugar exists in the system, the more it is taken by the cells of the body.

As emerging from the above study, cancer treatment protocols nowadays are aiming to control blood sugar levels in numerous ways. Physicians often suggest a healthy low-sugar diet, physical activity and drug administration in individuals suffering from cancer.

Sugar and Its Connection with Mental Health

Besides sugar bearing an impact on various physical functions of our system, it also affects mental health. Numerous trials examining sugar and its connection to the worsening of mental health disorders have been conducted by Malcolm Peet, an established and renowned mental health/psychiatry researcher. Dr.

Peet found a definite connection between high sugar intake and mental health disorder through extensive trials and studies on patients suffering from schizophrenia. Based on the outcomes of his studies, there is a clear association between elevated glucose levels and high risk of developing mental health problems like depression and schizophrenia.

Sugar has a detrimental effect on the central nervous system and mental health as a result. It actually downgrades mental activity by hindering the function of an important growth hormone called "BDNF", which leads to various chemical responses in the system that ultimately trigger long-term inflammation. The inflammation process hinders the activity of the immune system and leads to mental/brain issues. With BDNF, when amounts of this hormone fall to below physiological ranges, there is a higher risk of developing depression or schizophrenia.

Through extended and in-depth studies, Dr. Peet discovered that long-term inflammation in the system is triggered by high intake of sugar, which suppresses the normal activity of the immune system and makes it lose its power to fight back. Additional evidence from studies also validates the connection between high sugar consumption and aggravation of mental health disorders.

There are several studies featured in the British Journal Of Psychiatry that demonstrate a connection between diets high in sugar and mental health issues like stress, anxiety, depression, and others. These trials didn't concentrate on issues triggered by inflammation, but demonstrated instead that people who take high amounts of sugar on a regular basis are more likely to develop anxiety, depression, and other mental health disorders. Sugar-rich and carb-laden foods can also interfere with the neurotransmitters that help keep our moods stable. Consuming sugar stimulates the release of the mood-boosting neurotransmitter serotonin. Constantly over-activating these serotonin pathways can deplete our limited supplies of the neurotransmitter, which can contribute to symptoms of depression.

Additionally, sugar leads to a fast spike in adrenaline levels which triggers episodes of induced stress, anxiety, hyperactivity, and struggle to maintain focus. Scientists have revealed that following a diet that's nutrient-dense and low in sugar balanced mood levels and our ability to concentrate. People who took whole foods as a part of their diet regimes, were shown to experience better mood and deal with stressful situations more efficiently.

The Impact of Sugar on Our Kids

Sadly, sugar has been shown to be a contributing factor to high rates of child obesity and other health problems arising from high sugar intake. Child health experts across the world are worried that excessive sugar intake in children's diets is damaging to their health. Its high consumption can lead to an increased gain of body fat and raises the risk of childhood obesity.

Based on Baylor University of Texas studies and trials, the heightened tendency of childhood obesity rates over the past years is clearly associated with a high intake of sugar by kids over the same timeframe. We can't neglect the reality that our kids take excessive amounts of sugar and eventually can become obese. The majority of sugar intake originates from candy, breakfast cereals, sweetened granola bars, processed juices, and fizzy drinks.

The childhood obesity rates are consistently rising every year with our children suffering from poor health. Pediatricians sadly reveal that now, more than ever, children are treated for health problems that used to only bother adults mostly in the past such as elevated blood pressure, heart problems, and diabetes. All these conditions are associated with a high sugar intake.

Sugar Addictive Attributes in Relation to the Brain

It's easy to see how we can get hooked on sugar. When a person consumes sugar, just like any food, it activates the tongue's taste receptors. Then, signals are sent to the brain, lighting up reward pathways and causing a surge of feel-good hormones to be released. Animal trials demonstrated changes in the dopamine levels of the brain after the intake of sugar. Sugar "hijacks the brain's reward pathway," neuroscientist Jordan Gaines Lewis explained. While stimulating the brain's reward system with a piece of chocolate now and then is pleasurable and probably harmless, when the reward system is activated too much and too frequently, we start to run into problems. Over-activating this reward system kickstarts a series of unfortunate events — loss of control, cravings, and increased tolerance to sugar.

You may even call being hooked on sugar an 'addiction'. Some experts say consuming sugar produces effects similar to that of cocaine, by altering mood possibly through its ability to induce reward and pleasure, leading the person to seek out more sugar. While people who frequently eat sugar do not experience the tremor and chills or harsh withdrawals drug addicts experience when they withdraw the use of drugs, people do experience strong cravings for sugar. The reality is that quite simply the brain's rewards system and the circuits that control eating behavior are the same ones that respond to substances of addiction.

Be Cautious of Concealed Sugars

Studies conducted by University of Vermont's nutrition department found out that only a small minority of Americans actually comply with the standard guideline of taking no more than 150 calories from sugar daily. This guideline has been published by the AHA (American Heart Association), and functions as a target for individuals to meet by decreasing their sugar intake daily.

Sugar is sneakily hidden in so many kinds of foods that you will have to read every food label carefully in order to monitor your sugar consumption. Many food labels, however, are often misleading or ambiguous about containing sugar. There are two general rules when it comes to deciphering food labels:

No 1: Look for any words ending in -ose e.g sucralose, fructose, dextrose,e tc.

No 2: Pay close attention to names like "evaporated cane sugar" or "evaporated cane juice".

Any foods containing those should be limited. Furthermore, high fructose corn syrup is a a big no no. These sugars commonly found in foods are highly processed sugar which may lead to various health problems when taken excessively.

The most common offender in a person's diet isn't sweets but soft drinks/sodas. These include soda, lemonades, ice tea, juice cocktails, and other drinks with a high sugar content.

A single can of soda contains the equivalent of 10 teaspoons of sugar. This amount of sugar, especially in liquid form, skyrockets the blood sugar and causes an insulin reaction in the body. Over time, this can lead to diabetes or insulin resistance, not to mention weight gain and other health problems. Soft drink companies are the largest user of sugar in the country.

What is in Soda?

Phosphoric Acid: Soda contains phosphoric acid, which interferes with the body's ability to absorb calcium and can lead to osteoporosis, cavities, and bone softening. Phosphoric Acid also interacts with stomach acid, slowing digestion and blocking nutrient absorption.

Artificial Sweeteners: In diet sodas, aspartame is used as a substitute for sugar, and can actually be more harmful. It has been linked to different health problems including seizures, multiple sclerosis, brain tumors, diabetes, and emotional disorders. It converts to methanol at warm temperatures and methanol breaks down to formaldehyde and formic acid. Diet sodas also increase the risk of metabolic syndrome, which causes belly fat, high blood sugar, and raised cholesterol.

Caffeine: Most sodas contain caffeine, which has been linked to certain cancers, breast lumps, irregular heartbeat, high blood pressure, and other problems.

The Water: The water used in soda is just simple tap water and can contain chemicals like chlorine, fluoride, and traces of heavy metals.

Obesity: Harvard researchers have recently positively linked soft drinks to obesity. The study found that 12-year-olds who drank soda were more likely to be obese than those who didn't, and for each serving of soda consumed daily, the risk of obesity increased 1.6 times.

Lack of Nutrients: There is absolutely no nutritional value in soda whatsoever. Not only are there many harmful effects of soda, but there are not even any positive benefits to outweigh them. Soda is an unnatural substance that harms the body.

Ways To Cut Down On Sugar

Making a few adjustments to your diet can help you cut down on unnecessary sugar consumption:

Reduce the sugar you add to hot drinks. Do so gradually to give your tastebuds time to adjust. Try adding a sprinkle of cinnamon to cappuccino or hot chocolate. Cinnamon has several health benefits and adds flavor without the sweetness.

Avoid low-fat 'diet' foods which tend to be high in sugars. Instead, have smaller portions of the regular versions.

Be wary of 'sugar-free' foods. These often contain artificial sweeteners like sucralose, saccharin, and aspartame. Although these taste sweet, research suggests that they don't help curb a sweet tooth so they tend to send confusing messages to the brain and that can lead to over-eating.

Balance your carb intake with protein like fish, chicken, and turkey. Foods high in protein slow stomach emptying which helps manage cravings.

Swap white bread, rice, and pasta for other versions like oats, quinoa, brown and wild rice and pasta, zoodles, and cauliflower rice.

Reduce the sugar in recipes and add spices to boost flavor and taste.

Enjoy herbal teas or water with slices of citrus fruits for flavoring instead of juice or soda.

For a pick-me-up, have a piece of whole fruit with a handful of nuts or a small tub of non dairy yogurt. Both contain protein which helps balance blood sugar and energy levels.

Right behind soft drinks/sodas are processed foods. Both of these should be eliminated when focusing on a healthier and cleaner diet. Drinking plain water or unsweetened tea in the place of soft drinks and eating natural whole foods instead of processed food is a great start for cleansing our diet and bodies.

Chapter 10

Inflammatory Syndrome – How to Counteract the Effects of this Silent Killer

Battling a New Epidemic

The term "inflammation", is basically an immune reaction triggered by our systems to prevent any infection by bacteria or damage from injuries. If we examine human history itself, we will find that there were bacterial disorders that were widespread, affecting a large part of the population. However, somehow, they eventually diminished and posed very little threat. Some of these past disorders include smallpox, influenza, typhoid fever, and bubonic plague, which are almost extinct today.

While the majority of the above bacterial illnesses have almost vanished, today we are facing an entirely different epidemic. These include health problems that dimish your quality of life and well-being such as breathing problems, Alzheimer's, allergies, autoimmune disorders, skin problems, and many more. All these issues that plague people all over the world, especially the Western population aren't caused by bacteria like in the past but are mostly likely stemming from inflammation.

In the past two decades, the frequency of degenerative diseases has been constantly on the rise. Researchers have found that inflammatory disorders have been affecting Americans at an alarming rate because of poor diet habits and increased levels of stress and anxiety. Without any substantial changes to our diet and lifestyle patterns, the country will keep on suffering from diseases that most likely have underlying inflammatory cause.

What Are The Effects of Inflammation on the System?

When we use the word "inflammation", we usually think of symptoms like "heat", "high temperature", "Irritation", "swelling" and pain somewhere. When a lesion or cut gets inflamed, we can see the inflammation with our own eyes. However, inflammation is not always externally visible like that. The physical signs of "hidden" inflammation can be visible but at a much later stage, often times whenit's too late.

Chronic inflammation can lead to a variety of issues that can lead to a decline in health, as well as possible accelerated aging.

Disorders Triggered By Inflammation

There are various health issues connected with inflammation. Some of the most commonly emerging ones are different kinds of arthritis. Arthritis is a broad term that refers to inflammation in the joint area. Some of the most frequent/common kinds of inflammation-triggered arthritis or arthritis related problems are:

- Rheumatoid arthritis

- Polymyalgia Rheumatica

- Bursitis

- Shoulder Tendinitis

- Gouty Arthritis

Other problems targeting the bones and joints of our body may possibly be contributed to inflammation are:

- Osteoarthritis

- Fibromyalgia

- Neck and back pain

Shockingly enough, the World Health Organization reveals that over 13 millions of people annually lose their lives from cardiovascular disorders. It has been found that heart disease and related disorders may be caused by chronic inflammation. Based on *National Institute of Health* findings, inflammation is a crucial factor for the development of heart disease and its aggravation.

In order to lessen the likelihood of developing such disorders, we must, as a society, adopt a healthier diet and lifestyle.

Foods That Lead To Inflammation

For those affected by inflammation, diets rich in carbs and low in protein intake can be destructive. It has be hypothesized that high carb and low protein diets lead to inflammation while the opposite diet (low carbs/high protein intake), actually keeps inflammation under control and all the negative side effects connected to it.

Every individual person is different, and thus it is important to recognize how certain foods affect YOU. What might be inflammatory for one person, may not be inflammatory for you and vice versa. We suggest keeping a food journal to find out what foods work for you.

Processed sugars and foods with an elevated Glycemic Index (G.I) raise insulin levels and trigger an immune system response. There is a communication between inflammatory mediators (prostaglandins, cytokines), and insulin or blood sugar amounts. It is shown that insulin can trigger an inflammatory reaction within the system.

Some of the worst foods that trigger an inflammatory response in the body are:

No 1: Sugar/Sweets. High amounts of sugar consumption have been associated with weight issues, inflammation, and diabetes.

No 2: Common vegetable oils for cooking and baking such as corn, soy, vegetable. Oils with a high omega-6 fatty acid/low omega-3 acid ratio can also lead to inflammation.

No 3: Trans fats. These fats are typically found in junk food/fast food meals. They are also associated with inflammation, resistance to insulin, and other chronic disorders.

No 4: Milk and dairy products. Dairy products can also result in inflammation in many people,, especially in the female population, due to the hormones and to the fact that it is highly allergenic.

No 5: Red or processed meat. Eating red and processed meat e.g corned beef and hot dogs, is also associated with immune reactions that lead to chronic inflammation within our systems. There is also a connection between processed meat consumption and cancer risk.

Other types of foods suspect of causing inflammation are grains/flour which contain gluten, alcohol, synthetic food preservatives, and grain-fed meats. All the above foods should be avoided as much as possible.

Link between Stress and Inflammation

Chronic emotional, mental, and physical stress can trigger inflammation. When the system is exposed to stress of any kind, cortisol levels start to rise within the body.

Cortisol is a steroid hormone that is produced in response to high levels of stress. This may occur from real stressful events that you are aware of or can be a result of an unhealthy diet or lifestyle causing physical stress that you may not be aware of. This causes your stress fight or flight response, which is usually a short term response, to not be switched off, which can lead to a chronic inflammatory state.

In fact, chronic stress has a negative impact on various bodily functions. It raises blood pressure and chronic high blood pressure also puts blood vessels under a tremendous amount of stress. Strokes and heart failures are a common phenomenon in people suffering from chronic stress because of the chronic inflammatory responses being triggered non-stop.

It is vital to learn ways to deal with high stress levels so that you avoid chronic inflammation.

Some valuable relaxation methods include:

- Mild exercise

- Yoga/Meditation

- Learning ways to keep emotional tranquility

- Breathing exercises

- Tai Chi

How to Treat Inflammation

The traditional and common treatment of inflammation is the prescription of anti-inflammatory pills. The most typically administered drugs in this case are those that provide relief from pain (pain-relievers).

Not long ago, the *American Geriatrics Society* has taken off nearly all non-steroidal and anti-inflammatory drugs from their guide of suggested drugs for people 75+ who experience chronic pain. It was found out that these drugs are overly prescribed, much more than necessary, and this may lead to negative side effects on the health of older people. Researchers have found that commonly used pain-relievers like ibuprofen, naproxen, and aspirin are not really beneficial for those going through chronic pain.

Anti-inflammatory drugs aim to lessen pain and discomfort, minimize swelling, and control inflammation symptoms. They are speculated to help with the development of inflammatory disorder, but they don't always function as intended. Anti-inflammatory substances for pain relief feature NSAIDS such as Ibuprofen and Aspirin. Other substances are the ones called corticosteroids (cortisone, prednisone).

Typically, anti-inflammatory drug substances have many side effects. For instance, the use of cortisone for extended periods of time can lead to serious problems with bone strength and integrity. Many chronic takers of NSAIDS also develop stomach ulcers and internal bleeding and the gastric wall is further exposed to stomach acid in those who consume NSAIDS for longer periods of time to fight inflammation.

Alternative medicine methods approach the matter of inflammation from another perspective. Instead of prescribing synthetic drugs to hinder inflammatory reactions, they suggest using the power of diet, targeted supplements, and lifestyle changes. Alternative medicine adopts a more natural way of treatment as opposed to taking artificial drugs, but the trick is trying to pinpoint the exact cause of inflammation.

It isn't beneficial to only treat the symptoms, but it's just as important to pinpoint the leading culprit of said inflammation.

Inflammation Testing-Blood Examination

In those who suffer from long-term inflammation, there is an existing protein secreted by the inflamed region that travels through the bloodstream. One of the most common blood tests to find out inflammation is CRP (C-reactive protein test). This test can pinpoint any heightened levels of the protein, which is considered a sign of inflammation.

In several situations when an individual suffers from chronic inflammation which leads to a serious disorder like heart disease, or connective tissue (muscle, joints, bones, ligaments) disease, the CRP levels are elevated. These levels are precisely detected through blood testing.

Homocysteine amounts in the blood can also be determined from blood testing. Homocysteine is an acid that is produced by the system physiologically when we consume excessive amounts of red meat. When homocysteine levels are abnormally elevated, the person is at a high risk of developing heart problems, atherosclerosis, heart failure, stroke and even Alzheimer's disease.

What's the Key Culprit of Inflammation?

Researchers and medical experts keep on examining the leading cause of inflammation. With so many contributing factors and issues linked to our diets, it's no surprise that gut inflammation plays a vital role in inflammation.

Leaky Gut Syndrome may be the leading cause of many digestive tract diseases like IBS, Crohn's Syndrome, and celiac disease. When someone has a leaky gut, foreign substances from digested food can leak into the blood stream where it can be treated as a foreign invader, triggering an immune response. This can trigger the onset of various inflammatory disorders like food and other allergies, arthritis, and any variety of autoimmune disorders.

Not only can a leaky gut trigger autoimmune issues and digestive issues, it has been suggested recently that it may contribute to cognitive issues such as brain fog and memory issues as well.

Treating symptoms of the problem is akin to patching a leak with a piece of tape. Sure, it may help temporarily but it doesn't solve the problem. Finding the root cause of why your body is in a state of chronic inflammation is vital when you wish to attain good health.

Chapter 11

Spinal Degeneration

Unless you've been living under a rock, chances are you probably know someone with degenerative joint disease (DJD) also known as osteoarthritis. About 27 million Americans over the age of 25 have DJD, while 34% of those over 65 have DJD. As this is more common among the elderly, we can expect these numbers to continue to rise as the proportion of Americans over 65 grows.

What Is a Degenerative Joint Disease (DJD)?

The degenerative joint disease is a progressive disease that attacks the cartilage of the body, the hard tissue that covers the ends of the bones and joints so that the bones can move smoothly. DJD is considered the most common form of arthritis and is the leading cause of adult joint pain, affecting mostly the elderly and worsening as we age..

The terms degenerative arthropathy, degenerative arthritis and osteoarthritis are often used interchangeably. All are essentially the same type of disorder that over time causes the cartilage to wear out and cause pain in process. Osteoarthritis tends to worsen over time with more wear and tear and unfortunately, there is no cure.

You can develop osteoarthritis symptoms throughout the body, but it most often affects the neck, the lower back, the knees, the hips, the shoulders, and the fingers. Symptoms can include, but not limited to:

- Intermittent joint pain

- Stiffness (especially in the morning after getting up)

- Difficulty in tasks of daily living such a squatting, bending, walking up stairs, etc

- When DJD affects your hips, you may feel pain in the groin, thighs, buttocks or knees.

- When DJD affects the joints in your hands, your fingers can become enlarged, injured, hardened and numb

- DJD in the spine can cause numbness in the neck and a stiff lower back

- Grinding in your joints

Natural Treatment of Degenerative Joint Disease / Osteoarthritis

Although it is not possible to completely cure degenerative joint disease, there are many natural treatment options for osteoarthritis that can have a great effect on pain and the quality of life. These include exercising and staying active, avoiding weight gain and maintaining a healthy weight, an anti-inflammatory diet, chiropractic care, saunas, and massage therapy to name a few.

Essentially, this all helps to reduce the severity of the symptoms and delay the progression of the disease to prevent more cartilage loss.

The main objectives of all degenerative diseases/osteoarthritis treatment are to relieve inflammation/swelling, to control pain, and to improve mobility and joint function.

Stay Active

While most people with osteoarthritis typically have joint pain and limited mobility, many find that they feel better and generally experience fewer symptoms when they are active. In fact, exercise is considered one of the most important treatments for degenerative joint disease. Exercise is important to reduce inflammation, increase blood flow,, increase flexibility, strengthen muscles (including the heart), and to maintain a healthy body weight. Regular exercise is an effective way to improve mood, relieve stress and control stress hormones such as cortisol, and help you sleep better.

Since each DJD patient differs in terms of physical performance and pain perception, the exercise program will depend on the specific condition of each person and the stability of the joints. The ideal exercise program should include:

- Strengthening exercises to improve muscle strength, which supports the affected joints

- Aerobic activities to improve blood pressure, circulation and inflammation

- Agility activities to keep your joints flexible and supportive with daily activities

Exercise programs should start slowly and although you may feel soreness afterwards, it should not be very painful.

Reduce Inflammation and Support the Cartilage with a Nutrient-Rich Diet

Research indicates that poor nutrition can increase inflammation and increase enzymes that can destroy collagen and other important proteins required to maintain healthy tissue.

One of the ways in which you can help your body maintain valuable cartilage and reduce inflammation include the use of all types of natural anti-inflammatory foods. These provide essential fatty acids, antioxidants, minerals and vitamins that support the immune system, relieve pain, and contribute to the healthy formation of tissue and bone.

Your diet should be well rounded and consists of:

- Fresh vegetables (all types): Eat the rainbow! This should be the majority of what you eat. Avoid nightshade vegetables such as tomatoes, potatoes, peppers, and eggplant as they can increase inflammation

- Whole fruit: They are a great source of vitamins and antioxidants.

- Herbs, spices, and teas: Many are anti-inflammatory

- Probiotic foods: non dairy yogurt, kombucha, sauerkraut helps with gut health which is good for the immune system and for absorption of vitamins and minerals

- Wild fish, eggs from pasture raised poultry, and grass fed meat: contains higher levels of omega 3 fatty acid which helps with decreasing inflammation. Their farmed and conventionally grain fed counterparts can actually cause more inflammation.

- Healthy fats: grass-fed butter, coconut oil, extra virgin olive oil, nuts/seeds

- Bone broth: contains collagen and helps to maintain healthy joints

Your diet should limit or eliminate foods that promote inflammation such as:

- Refined vegetable oils: such as rapeseed oil, corn and soybean oil, 'vegetable' oil which are all high in inflammatory omega 6 fatty acids

- Pasteurized dairy products (a common allergen) and conventional meat, poultry and eggs, which also contain hormones, antibiotics and omega-6 fatty acids that contribute to inflammation

- Refined carbohydrates, sugary sweets, soda, and processed foods all can trigger inflammation because they are high in sugars and chemicals

- Trans fat / hydrogenated fats

Maintain a Healthy Body Weight

Having excess weight causes increased pressure on the degenerated joints, increasing symptoms in the process. Patients with DJD should try to maintain a healthy body weight in order to not only relieve symptoms, but to keep their DJD from worsening. This should be done through healthy long term lifestyle changes and not calorie restriction as that can actually cause nutritional deficits that are harmful to the healing process.

Get Enough Rest / Relaxation

With today's fast paced society, many of us do not have enough hours in a day to get what we need to get done. This tends to lead to late nights and increased stress, with us sacrificing our sleep and rest in the process. Unfortunately, the lack of rest and sleep can be detrimental to your health in the long run because not only can it contribute to hormonal imbalances and weight gain, your body may also have a difficult time repairing tissues throughout the body, making it difficult to heal. When you are chronically stressed, your body remains in a fight or flight state, it is difficult to keep inflammation to a minimum. Everyone is different and will have different requirements of what constitutes enough sleep but we should all aim to be in bed before 10 pm. We should all also incorporate relaxation techniques into our daily routine, such a meditation, deep breathing, yoga, or tai chi to name a few.

Control the Pain Naturally

Dealing with pain can be one of the most difficult tasks in the fight against degenerative joint disease because it undermines the quality of life, the ability to do good work, and independence. Many doctors prescribe non-steroidal anti-inflammatory drugs (NSAIDs included) or even surgery to relieve pain when the situation becomes severe enough, but there are many other things to try first. Some of the most popular complementary therapies and alternatives that fight pain are:

- **Acupuncture:** Studies show that patients who receive acupuncture usually have less pain than patients in control groups. It has been shown that acupuncture relieves the symptoms of back and neck pain, muscle pain and joint stiffness, osteoarthritis and chronic headache.

- **Massage Therapy:** A professional massage can help to improve blood circulation, bring blood to sensitive areas, relax the mind and relieve stress.

- **Foot Reflexology:** For centuries foot reflexology has been used to stimulate the nervous system and help the body with stress, fatigue, pain and emotional problems.

- **Homeopathy and Essential Oils:** There are many homeopathic remedies and essential oils that have been used for pain and inflammation throughout history such as arnica and peppermint oil. It is important to research how to use these correctly because even though they are natural, they have the ability to cause issues if used incorrectly.

What Are The Causes of Osteoarthritis / DJD?

People with DJD often do not have enough healthy cartilage as they get older which often leads to pain as there is no longer a buffer between moving bones. We need cartilage so that the bone "slides" and absorbs the vibrations or shocks that we experience with everyday movement.

When the disease has progressed, the bones rub together in a manner that causes inflammation, swelling, pain, loss of flexibility and sometimes changes in joint shape.

In severe cases of the degenerative joint disease, small bone deposits called osteophytes, sometimes called spurs, can also form on the edges of the joints. The main problem with bone spurs is that they can break off into the joint space, causing more pain and inflammation.

Risk Factors for Degenerative Joint Disease

The cause of DJD is not completely known at this time but there are some factors that increases a person's risk for developing DJD. That includes:

- Age: the elderly have a higher occurrence but it can occur at any age.

- Sex: More men have DJD younger than 45 years old but women are the main ones that have it over 45 years of age.

- Overweight or obese

- Suffer from joint injuries that lead to malformations

- Work or hobby that requires repeated movements

- Having certain genetic defects that affect the development of cartilage and collagen in the joints

- Have DJD in your family

Do not confuse osteoarthritis (DJD) and rheumatoid arthritis. Rheumatoid arthritis is the second most common form of arthritis after osteoarthritis. It is considered an autoimmune disease because the immune system attacks healthy body tissues that make up the joints. Osteoarthritis is caused by mechanical wear and tear of the joints and is not classified as an autoimmune disease.

DJD and RA both produce pain, swelling, and, over time, joint damage or malformations. Compared to RA, DJD usually starts later in life where as rheumatoid arthritis can occur early in life and usually causes symptoms other than joint/cartilage tissue loss, including fatigue, decreased immunity, changes in the skin tissue, lungs and eyes or blood vessels.

Summary of Degenerative Joint Disease:

- Degenerative joint disease, also known as osteoarthritis, is the leading type of arthritis in adults.

- DJD causes a reduction in cartilage and joint tissue that causes joint pain, swelling and problems with mobility of the joint.

- It can caused by a combination of factors including genetics, severe inflammation, poor diet, repetitive movements and aging ("normal wear" of the body).

You may be able to prevent DJD by eating a nutritious diet and staying active and can relieve the pain from DJD by using alternative treatments such as acupuncture, massage, and heat treatments.

Chapter 12

Decompression for Spinal Problems

What Is Decompression Therapy?

Decompression therapy is a non surgical manipulation of the spine used to relieve pain and improve spinal function. It involves stretching the spine with the use of a traction table or any other motorised device that may be similar to it. The procedure is non invasive and is usually carried out by a chiropractor, a trained and licensed medical expert who specialises in mechanical manipulation of the bone and joints.

Decompression therapy is a ground-breaking treatment that involves the careful and precisely measured mechanical stretching of the spine which is a gentle, graded approach to providing relief to disc- related pain and to stimulate blood and oxygen flow through the spine, enabling the lubrication of the discs and providing long term improvement of symptoms in patients with chronic neck and back pain.

Spinal decompression is performed on a computer controlled traction table. It operates under the same basic principles that chiropractors have been using over the years to stretch the spine and provide effective relief from painful symptoms. This therapy works by slowly and steadily stretching the spinal column to remove the abnormal pressure that had been exerted on the discs that sit between the vertebrae. This stretching action in turn creates a negative pressure inside the discs in the spine that helps to draw protruding disc material ('bulging disc' or 'slipped disc') back into place. The stretching also promotes increased blood flow into spinal discs, bringing in nutrient rich fluids and oxygen which in turn promotes cell renewal and tissue repair.[4]

Who Discovered Decompression Therapy?

Decompression therapy is NOT a new technology and has been around for over 30 years. In 1985, Allan Dyer discovered decompression therapy and six years after, he developed VAX-D, the first decompression table. The original VAX-D decompression table was controlled by a pneumatic system that gradually pulled and released with traction and was applied to the back or legs to reduce muscle spasm.[2] Today, this revolutionary technology is computer-aided and is FDA-approved. The treatment process is safe and usually lasts for a period of thirty to forty minutes per treatment session. A typical spinal decompression treatment protocol consists of about 12-20 sessions over four to six weeks. However, some conditions may require lesser or more visits depending on the severity of the condition.

The Science behind Decompression Therapy

The main theory behind decompression therapy is when traction is provided to compressed structures in the spine, both pressure and pain are relieved in the affected regions. In decompression therapy, the aim is to relieve pain and promote an optimal environment for healing in conditions such as herniated discs, bulging discs or degenerating discs.

A herniated, protruded, bulging, or slipped disc refers to a condition that occurs when disc material from the disc's inner core leak out from where it is usually confined. This can cause pain, swelling and discomfort in the back and if the disc material pinch, inflame or irritate a nearby nerve, this can cause sharp and shooting pains that radiates to various parts of the body. Typically, a herniated disc occurs in the cervical spine (neck) or the lumbar spine (lower back region) with rare cases occurring in the thoracic spine (mid back region). It seems to be the most common in the lower back where most of the weight bearing occurs.

Because a herniated disc is, at its core, a structural problem, medications can only mask pain symptoms for a short period of time without actually providing treatment for the condition.

Why Decompression Therapy?

Non invasive spinal decompression therapy has often been a last resort for many over the years for those with neck and back pain. Patients with back pain usually first turn to NSAIDS or opioid pain medications only to discover that it only brings temporary relief with a long list of adverse side effects including liver and kidney impairment, not to mention the possibility of addiction with opioids. With decompression therapy, it is non invasive, does not require recovery time as surgery would, and does not have any of the side effects NSAIDs or opioids do.

The benefits of non invasive spinal decompression therapy may include:

- Relief of irritated nerve roots from the herniated discs, leading to a reduction of radiating symptoms including pain, numbness, and tingling in the extremities.
- Relief of pressure/pain in the spine in the area of the herniated discs
- May help retract the bulging disc material as well as improving blood flow and oxygen in the area to help with inflammation
- Can help stretch load bearing areas or areas that are compressed due to everyday activities and/or work.

Decompression therapy can fit neatly into your everyday routine, without any recovery time required and can have long lasting effects if the prescribed regimen is followed.

What to Expect With Decompression Therapy

People who have been living with persistent neck, back or sciatic nerve pain caused by herniated or degenerative spinal discs don't have to live a life dependent on medication or resort to surgery as non invasive spinal decompression therapy has shown to provide remarkable pain relief.

Decompression therapy is carried out on a motorized table controlled by a computer. Depending on which area of the body is being decompressed, belts and other equipment is used to stabilize certain parts of the body. For example, to treat a disc problem that affects the lower back, a harness is fitted comfortably around the hips and is attached to the lower end of the table near the feet. A specific program prescribed by your chiropractor is entered into the computer and the table gently and slowly slides back and forth in increments, lengthening the spine in the process.

A single decompression session lasts from 15 to 30 minutes. The average decompression treatment protocol consists of an average of twelve to twenty sessions lasting over a period of four to six weeks. Some patients experience relief after the first session; others do not until after several sessions. Dependent on the level of injury, some patients will need to start slowly and work their way into the program. Some may feel sore after a session, others will not. Everyone is different. If you have any questions about the protocol or concerns, please let your treatment team know. For long lasting relief, the entire treatment protocol should be followed.

Contraindications of Decompression Therapy

Despite the relative safety of non invasive spinal decompression therapy, there are patients who may not be a good candidate. Please speak with your treatment team if you:

- Are pregnant, as pregnant women are often plagued with back and sciatic pain.

- Have broken/collapsed/compressed vertebrae
- Had a spinal fusion surgery.
- Have existing spinal implants or artificial disc in the spine
- Had a history of back surgery
- Have been diagnosed with spinal osteoporosis

Is Decompression Therapy Right For Me?

Non invasive decompression therapy is a viable option for those who have been suffering from pain from herniated discs with or without nerve root involvement. It is not a new technology; it has been around for over 30 years and have been tried by many patients with success. The way decompression therapy works is by addressing the structural and physiological changes that occur with a herniated disc, something that pain medications are unable to do. With the right treatment protocol and adherence to that protocol, patients may be able to return to their life before injury without having to resort to surgery.

Chapter 13

The Mystery that is Neuropathy

Neuropathy (nerve damage) can be caused by various conditions, ranging from the most common cause, diabetes, to even treatment regimens like cancer chemotherapy. This condition is sometimes termed peripheral neuropathy and describes multiple health issues involving damage to the peripheral nerves and the symptoms associated with those disorders. Peripheral neuropathy can cause weakness, altered sensation and numbness in the hands and feet. It may also have an impact on other parts of your body. People usually describe the pain from peripheral neuropathy as sharp, burning, or tingling. Symptoms often get better, particularly when a curable disease causes them.

Unfortunately, neuropathic pain is a difficult condition to manage. In a large percentage of patients, current treatment techniques fail to provide adequate or tolerable pain relief. Inadequate diagnosis and a lack of knowledge of the processes involved, poor care of concomitant diseases, incorrect understanding or selection of treatment choices, and the use of unsuitable outcomes measurements are the four primary reasons why therapies for neuropathic pain fail.

Causes

Peripheral neuropathy is nerve damage produced by a variety of diseases rather than being a single illness. Peripheral neuropathy can be caused by many different health conditions and symptoms might range from moderate to severe, although they are seldom fatal. They might appear for days, weeks, or years and may improve on their own in some situations, necessitating no further treatment. Peripheral nerve cells, unlike nerve cells in the central nervous system, continue to develop throughout life.

In mononeuropathy, only one nerve is damaged. Multiple mononeuropathy, also known as mononeuropathy multiplex, is a kind of neuropathy that affects two or more nerves in separate anatomical locations. Polyneuropathy is when many, if not all, of the nerves in one area are damaged.

Diabetes is the most common cause of peripheral neuropathy. The other common causes are idiopathic (spontaneous or unknown cause), HIV-related, chemotherapy-related, and autoimmune-related. Autoimmune illnesses are a common cause of peripheral neuropathy. This type of disease occurs when the immune system attacks itself. Some examples include Sjogren's syndrome, lupus, rheumatoid arthritis, Guillain-Barre syndrome, chronic inflammatory demyelinating polyneuropathy, and vasculitis.

What Role Does Diabetes Play in Causing Neuropathy?

Nerve issues might occur at any time in a person living with diabetes. Neuropathy is sometimes the first indication of diabetes. The longer the duration a person lives with diabetes, the more likely a neuropathy will develop. Neuropathy affects around half of all diabetics.

Although the specific causes of diabetic neuropathy are unknown, a number of variables may play a role, including:

High blood sugar: High blood glucose damages nerve cells by causing chemical changes that impede their capacity to send impulses. It can also harm the blood arteries that supply the neurons with oxygen and nourishment.

Metabolic factors: High triglyceride and cholesterol levels, in addition to glucose levels, are linked to an increased risk of neuropathy. Neuropathy is more likely to present in people who are overweight or obese.

Genetic Factors: Some hereditary characteristics may predispose some people to nerve illness more than others.

According to a major American research, 47% of people with diabetes have some form of peripheral neuropathy. At the time of a diabetes diagnosis, neuropathy is predicted to be already present in 7.5% of patients. Distal symmetric polyneuropathy accounts for more than half of all cases.

Prevalence of Peripheral Neuropathy in the United States

To acquire a clearer picture of the peripheral neuropathy prevalence in the US, it makes sense to categorize incidence according to cause.

Diabetic Neuropathy

The diagnosis of diabetic peripheral neuropathy is based on both clinical indicators and quantitative tests, and it may exist despite the absence of symptoms. Peripheral neuropathy affects 28% of individuals with diabetes in the United States. In a survey of 4400 Belgian patients, researchers discovered that 7.5% already had neuropathy before they were diagnosed with diabetes. After 25 years, the percentage of people with neuropathy had risen to 45%. Diabetic neuropathy is prevalent among the hospital clinic population in the United Kingdom, with a frequency of about 29%.

Diabetic peripheral neuropathy can have profound implications. Diabetes mellitus significantly increases the risk of lower limb amputation, with around 50% of diabetics developing a foot ulcer over their lifespan. Furthermore, neuropathic pain and reduced sensation can lead to various negative consequences, including falls, lower quality of life, limitations in daily activities, and symptoms of depression.

HIV-Associated Sensory Peripheral Neuropathy

The most frequent neurological consequence of HIV infection is peripheral neuropathy. Despite this, it is underdiagnosed and undertreated. The most prevalent kind of HIV neuropathy is sensory neuropathy (HIV-SN), which affects up to two-thirds of individuals with advanced illness in some situations.

Postherpetic Neuralgia (PHN)

PHN is a form of neuropathy caused by the reactivation of the herpes zoster virus. The virus persists in an inactive state within the spinal cord until the patient's immune response deteriorates due to aging, HIV infection, cancer, or immunosuppressive treatment, at which point it can reactivate.

According to data from *Clinical Infectious Diseases,* the total incidence rate of PHN was 57.5 cases per 100,000 person. Researchers also discovered that the proportion of people with herpes zoster who acquired PHN increased from 2007 to 2018 compared to 1994 to 2006.

Chemotherapy-Induced Peripheral Neuropathy (CIPN)

This is the most prevalent neurological complication of cancer therapy. It is a chemotherapy-related side effect that is dose-dependent. The pain and numbness in patients with CIPN are described as symmetric with a "glove and stocking" distribution.

The majority of individuals get neuropathic symptoms within six months after starting chemotherapy. As the treatment continues, the symptoms may increase. In many situations, once the therapy is stopped, it improves but may not completely resolve.

Chronic Inflammatory Demyelinating Polyradiculo neuropathy (CIDP)

CIDP (classified as an acquired idiopathic demyelinating neuropathy with a progressive phase > eight weeks) has relatively limited epidemiological data. It's definitely a rare illness, but the neurophysiological and nerve biopsy tests needed to detect it are complex. Thus, it's likely underdiagnosed. There are currently no accurate population estimates of its prevalence. However, some data shows a frequency of at least 1 per 100 000 people.

Alcohol

People who abuse alcohol are more likely to develop peripheral nerve damage. The question of whether this is due to a direct toxic impact of alcohol or a chronic nutritional deficit has been debated for a long time. In the United States, it is believed that 25% to 66% of chronic alcoholics suffer from neuropathy; however, the real prevalence in the general population is unclear. The bulk of the patients were middle-class working males, and those who drank continuously were more impacted than those who drank episodically.

Traditional Avenues Associated with the Treatment of Neuropathy

There are a variety of therapies available to assist in alleviating symptoms and peripheral neuropathy. The phrase "traditional/conventional neuropathy therapy" refers to treatment methods that doctors have given for a long time. Physical therapy, surgery, and injections for increased nerve pressure are some of the most frequent therapies.

Medical Treatment

Over-the-counter non-steroidal anti-inflammatory medicines like ibuprofen and aspirin are examples of this regimen. Headaches, stomach discomfort, stomach ulcers, dizziness, and elevated blood pressure are all possible side effects. These medicines can assist with pain, but they may not be enough. More potent medications, such as antidepressants or anticonvulsants, may also be administered. However, these medications can come with many side effects including, but not limited to, dry mouth, headaches, sexual dysfunction, dizziness, tiredness, nausea, sleepiness, weight gain, vomiting, and constipation.

Surgical Treatment

Surgery or interventional treatments that seek to relieve pain by cutting or damaging nerves are usually ineffective because they exacerbate nerve injury, and the portions of the peripheral and central nervous systems above the incision frequently keep sending pain signals ("phantom pain"). These surgeries have mostly been superseded by more advanced and less harmful, non-invasive treatments.

Other Approaches to Treatment of Neuropathy

Low-Intensity Red Light

The Semmes-Weinstein 10-g monofilament is commonly used to diagnose diabetic peripheral neuropathy (SWM). Recent research suggests that treating diabetic individuals with monochromatic near infrared red energy (MIRE) can improve their foot sensitivity to the SWM. In individuals with diabetic peripheral neuropathy, pulsed infrared light treatment (PILT) has been proven to improve peripheral sensitivity.

Vibration Therapy

Whole-Body Vibration (WBV) training is a novel form of somatosensory stimulation (SSS) exercise that has gained popularity in sports training and rehabilitation over the past ten years. WBV improves physical strength and balance with time. The treatment modality was shown in a recent study to have an influence on the pain level of a diabetic patient with neuropathy.

Although peripheral neuropathy is thought to be progressive and permanent, the patient's (Michigan Diabetic Neuropathy Score) MDNS score decreased considerably during the WBV trials.

Though research is still in its early phases, combining WBV with other therapeutic treatment methods might be beneficial.

Nutrition

People with diabetic neuropathy should try to maintain the blood glucose levels recommended by their doctors. To do these, they need to avoid processed carbohydrates such as sweets, sugary beverages, etc. Instead, focus on portion control and carbohydrates derived from high-fiber whole grains. Vegetables, fruits, and lean meats are also excellent sources of energy and nourishment. These dietary precautions on their own may not cure or reverse current nerve damage, but they can help you avoid additional injury.

While changing your diet to a healthier, whole foods based way of eating instead of relying on processed foods will provide your body with improved nourishment, you may not be getting everything your body requires to function optimally. Unfortunately, our food is often grown on depleted soils and may not contain all the vitamins and minerals we need. In addition, we are accosted by toxins everyday in the form of pesticides, pollution, poor air quality indoor and out, and chemicals in our daily products which can hinder our body's ability to absorb everything it needs from foods or over tax our body to get rid of these toxins, using up its resources in the process. This is where supplementation comes into play.

Targeted supplementation can be highly beneficial as it can help support the body in replenishing on what it is lacking. In addition, specific supplements can also support processes of the body, such as helping with blood sugar control which many with peripheral neuropathy have trouble with. While supplements alone will not help you treat neuropathy, it can support the body by giving it enough resources to work with. However, over supplementing is not only not useful, it can also be detrimental. The key is only supplementing as necessary.

Exercise and Lifestyle Changes

Although many of the most frequent causes of peripheral neuropathy are incurable, it's essential to recognize that regular exercise can not only help avoid some of them but it's also been shown to help relieve some of the condition's most unpleasant symptoms. The major treatment method for type 2 diabetes patients is aerobic exercise. In addition to endurance training, diabetes type 2 patients are given segmental strength training of the primary muscle groups.

Other lifestyle modification strategies include proper foot care e.g by wearing well-fitted, padded shoes and minimizing pressure to areas like knees and elbow. These measures help to reduce pain and the risk of trauma. Smoking can obstruct blood flow and cause blood vessels to constrict. Cessation of smoking improves blood flow, and blood vessels become healthier. Massages and acupuncture are examples of might help patients relax and feel better. Essential oils, like chamomile and lavender, can assist in relieving pain and increasing blood flow throughout the body.

Patient Experience with Neuropathy in Practice

The primary symptoms of peripheral neuropathy that I have seen in practice is physical pain in the feet, hands, arms, back, and knees with numbness and tingling being the most common complaints. Often times, these patients have been misdiagnosed for many years before they received the diagnosis of peripheral neuropathy which contributes to a deterioration of function with high pain levels. The most common contributing factors are diabetes, chemotherapy, and alcohol related nerve damage. The nerve damage and relating symptoms often lead to additional problems such as requiring assistive devices to walk with some cases where the patient is wheelchair bound, alter gait, balance problems leading to multiple falls, and inability to use their hands for daily functional activities.

Treatment of peripheral neuropathy is a complex multifactorial process but with the right combination of therapies and lifestyle changes, patients can significantly improve their function and quality of life.

Chapter 14

Blending Chiropractic Care with Traditional Medicine

In a survey of people seeking alternative care, of all other methods, chiropractic is used most often. The majority of chiropractors recognize the value of combined health care treatments. Unfortunately the same respect is not reciprocated by the medical profession as a whole. While a portion of chiropractors feel that their own discipline can and should treat all different types of illnesses and injuries, most recognize the role of traditional and modern medical practices.

The philosophy, however, is a step by step approach to health care starting with the least invasive and gradually working, if necessary, toward more invasive and aggressive treatments. An example may be in the case of the patient with stomach ailments. If after receiving complete chiropractic care for the possible subluxation related to the stomach area, and there is no relief, then the patient may be referred to a gastroenterologist. If this same patient were to begin their care with the gastroenterologist, they may have walked out of that office with a prescription in hand to treat the symptoms of indigestion, never really exploring the cause of the symptoms.

There are more thorough doctors who do not automatically prescribe medication and explore the reasons behind the symptoms but unfortunately, they can be difficult to find.

The most invasive and least desirable of any treatment is, of course, surgery. That should be the absolute last resort after exhausting all options, which should include trying chiropractic. If the nerve signals to the abdomen area were blocked, they may be unable to communicate clearly to the acid producing stomach that it needed to regulate acid production, thus possibly causing stomach issues.

There are today, unfortunately, very few medical doctors who make referrals the other way around – from their offices to the chiropractor. That seems to be changing for the better with more and more chiropractors being invited to attend medical conferences and to write for medical journals. It is, perhaps, the role of patients and chiropractors alike to keep educating doctors on the benefits of the less invasive methods of chiropractic. Through word of mouth from my patients alone, I have been able to connect with a number of doctors, including neurosurgeons and neurologists, as well as dentists as well!

The Doctor-Patient Relationship

Any type of health examination is an extremely personal interaction. I'm sure you can envision the situation: two people who are meeting perhaps for the first time sit together in a room. One tells the other what kinds of activities they are involved in to break the ice, then starts talking about their body – where it hurts, what past illnesses they have had, any problems they have with normal functions of the body. Pretty personal stuff! And that is all before the physical examination!

Chiropractic care is similar to any other kind of medical care in the fact that there is complete confidentiality between doctor and patient. The similarities, however, end there. Chiropractic care is thorough and takes a deep dive into looking at the whole person. Chiropractors examine not only the specific aches and pains or illnesses, but the entire lifestyle, family situation, occupation, and concerns even outside the realm of your health because all of it contributes to overall health. There are few such physicians out there that take the time and care enough to learn about every aspect of the patient's life. With chiropractors, however, it is more the norm than the exception.

You will find that with regular visits that your chiropractic team practically will become family. Many of my patients return with their spouses, parents, children, and friends, making it a true "family" affair! We have seen moms through their pregnancies, to their newborn babies, to grandparents well into their golden years. We have seen patients go through moves, job changes, marriages, and starting families of their own!

In the insurance driven medical industry, it is probably not a common occurrence to know your medical team well because you usually have a limited time frame to summarize your ailment and for the doctor to do the examination. A patch, maybe a prescription for pills and a co-pay later, you are probably on your way until the next physical or ailment

What to Expect During Your Visit to the Chiropractor

If you are new to the world of chiropractic, you may be a little unsure about what to expect. Is there going to be some massage-like table slab where I lay down to have someone pound my back and crack my spine? Will it hurt? Is there anyone else in the room with me during an examination or adjustment? These are all very good questions that left unanswered could dissuade someone from visiting a chiropractor.

You may be surprised to know that a visit to the chiropractor is one of the most relaxing and comfortable type of health care visits.

When you enter the chiropractic office, you will be greeted by a warm receptionist who is ready to answer your questions and also to gather some information from you. You will complete some paperwork on your health history and what your main health concerns are.

In most instances, you will not have any kind of adjustment or manipulation to your spinal column on the very first visit. This is a time for gathering information, including a comprehensive medical history and for the chiropractor to really listen to what concerns you. It is a time to establish trust, answer any questions you may have, and discuss what possible therapy could benefit you.

You may also have x-rays taken to see what is actually occurring where we can't see, as well as a physical exam that contain mobility and function testing. After all the x rays and testing, a follow-up visit may be scheduled to allow the team time to review the x rays and come up with a plan of care. This also gives the patient time to formulate any questions that they may not asked during their first visit.

During the 2nd visit, the team will review their findings from the first visit and introduce a plan of care for the patient. Hopefully, that will be the beginning of the journey for the patient into the world of chiropractic care!

Made in the USA
Monee, IL
16 August 2021

74916244R00085